Sincerely,

Shanna

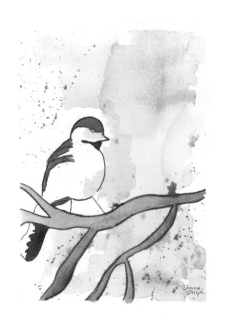

Sincerely, Shanna

How I Chose the Life I Wanted

A Memoir
Shanna Joseph

MILL CITY PRESS

Mill City Press, Inc.
2301 Lucien Way #415
Maitland, FL 32751
407.339.4217
www.millcitypress.net

Printed in the United States of America

ISBN-13: 978-1-6305-0456-4

Library of Congress Control Number: 2019921147

Dedicated to my husband, daughters, family and friends.

Sincerely,

Shanna

"Sincerely Shanna is an inspiring and empowering read for all those who want to love the life they live, to discover the secret to happiness and inner peace and to step onto the path of self-discovery. Although the author doesn't deny the physical and emotional aspects of her experience, she chooses to create a different reality—one that transcends the bounds of the illness and embraces the possibilities that come with shifting from fear to faith, from control to surrender, from turmoil to peace and from planning to living. She teaches us that nothing can stop us from living our lives when we have the courage to tap into the wisdom that exists within."

Linda Fallo-Mitchell, Ph.D., Intuitive Healer, Reiki Master, Editor of *Everyday Mystic: Finding the Extraordinary in the Ordinary*

"Sincerely Shanna is a real insight into the emotions of someone going through a life altering, extremely difficult journey while she faces her own mortality. Anyone can relate to trying to see what their body/mind/spirit needs are on their journeys- be it through cancer or another life altering experience. It gave a view into the real journey of someone trying to find the source of purpose, the life lived, where it has put them now, and how it is shaping their future."

Subuhee Hussain, MD. Hematology and Oncology

"I never paint dreams or nightmares.
I paint my own reality."

-Frida Kahlo

Prologue

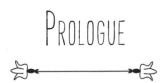

After the terrorist attacks of September 11th, I had a very strong premonition that I was going to get sick and die. Later, I thought that it was PTSD. It made sense after witnessing so many people fall to their deaths and barely getting out alive myself.

But why, I wondered, did I believe that I would get sick? Why didn't I believe that I would explode in another terrorist attack, die in a plane crash, or jump off a building like the rest of the 9/11 victims?

It was because deep inside I knew that there was a connection between being at Ground Zero and getting sick. However, it would take 10 years for my premonition to become a reality.

In those years, I visited countless ERs. A couple times I had a heart rate so fast that I thought I was having a heart attack. Other times I couldn't breathe. Sometimes my skin broke out in unexplained rashes. I felt lumps in my stomach and got MRIs to rule out abdominal disease. I had horrible headaches and visited a neurologist. I visited multiple hospitals with my husband with bizarre symptoms. But they could never find anything wrong with me.

And then finally, after my girls were born, I started to feel lumps in my breasts. Even though I was only in my 20s, I went for quarterly breast exams and sometimes biopsies at a top hospital in New York City. The results were always negative. 'Just extra tissue' they would say. 'Stress and high anxiety' I would hear over and over.

The sum of the medical visits was that many doctors in the New York area thought I was crazy.

But was I?

TABLE OF CONTENTS

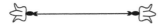

Dear Reader,

Sincerely, Shanna is a collection of letters that I wrote between 2012 and 2019 in a desperate search for meaning and happiness during the most challenging years of my life. Together they create a permanent catalog of the arduous and painful process that made writing them possible.

The letters reflect my up-and-down journey – like a ride on a roller coaster. Sometimes slow and steady, a long upward climb. Then a fast, scary descent into the depths of the earth, with the wind blowing through me and everything so blurry that I can't even see. A large pit in my stomach, nausea reaching from head to toe. Sometimes it steadies again, and I can almost enjoy the view. Other times we go straight up, around and around, and I know we will be going down again. I just don't know when.

In 2012, I was a 34-year-old woman who had "made it." I had an incredible family and lots of good friends, a high-powered financial marketing job in the heart of Manhattan, and a great house in an upscale suburban waterfront community. I was fit, healthy, still pretty, still smiling.

And I was a survivor. I had lived through 9/11, escaping from my office located directly across from the World Trade Center without a scratch, and, while heartbroken, alive, and with a greater appreciation for life.

I hadn't had many "big" problems in this first part of my life. A couple disappointments, but mostly successes and more successes.

Until, on November 12, 2012, after a decade of potential hypochondria, I found a lump in my breast when I was washing myself in the shower. It was near my armpit. I felt it again. Then I pinched it. I kept washing as if I hadn't felt it. Then I felt it again. I pinched it again. It was small but hard. There was no denying it: it was there.

On November 21, 2012, I was diagnosed with Stage 2 invasive ductal carcinoma breast cancer, and I completely fell apart. I wasn't equipped to deal with something like this and neither was anyone around me. Then on August 22, 2014, I received a Stage 4 diagnosis. It changed everything… forever.

Now I share the letters I wrote with you, dear reader, on my journey to acceptance.

This is not a cancer memoir. I know that because I have read many a cancer memoir. And many a cancer blog. I have read the stories about how the delicious routines of life were stolen from cancer patients. About the details of their PET scans, doctors' appointment, radiation procedures, and chemotherapy drips. About how there is still no cure. And not enough research dollars. About how we sit on couches, nauseous, tired, depressed, depleted. Waiting to die.

Unfortunately, those are real stories. I have lived many of them. And there is genuine uncertainty about whether my life will be cut short.

My cancer has progressed (grown) but is being controlled by modern science. I believe that this is the future of the disease. That there will be growing numbers of people like me. That our lifetimes will be prolonged, until one day the disease will be cured. This has enabled me to consider deeply what it means to live with my cancer, and not to die with it. My Present has become extended and long. Seven years and many progressions. I am still going.

Now I share the letters I wrote with you, dear reader, and how I chose to live the life I wanted.

So, let's begin the roller coaster ride.

Sincerely,
Shanna

KNOW YOURSELF AND YOUR BODY

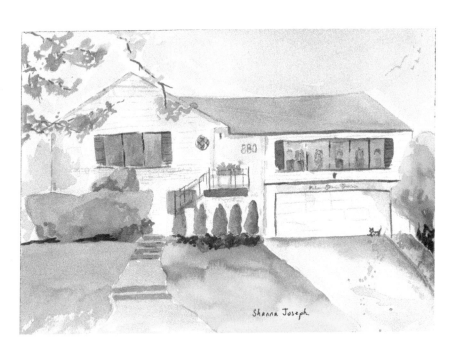

Shanna Joseph

Dear Family,

I will always be able to smell and feel what it was like to grow up with you in suburban Long Island, in that white split ranch, with the basketball hoop in the driveway and the play set in the backyard.

I remember lying for hours on that comforter on my bed with the curly pastel purple ribbons, book in hand, probably one from the Sweet Valley or Baby-Sitters Club series, at around age 10. There through the back window I can see the Elementary School. My music collection is piled high in the corner, and all around me my art masterpieces, including my self-portrait, hang carefully on the walls.

Mom, if I could step back in time, I know you would be cooking dinner, as usual – maybe chicken or steak, or spaghetti and meatballs, with some soggy veggies on the side. The TV is blaring, and pots and pans are strewn around the kitchen. The phone rings every couple of minutes so you and your friends can chat. You walk around the room with the long cord of the rotary phone dragging behind you, curling around and around until it is stuck in knots. "I'd better go," you say, with a small laugh and shake of your dark frizzy hair. You never say the word "goodbye."

After turning off the oven and waving the smoke away, you pile Dad's plate high with food. Then you cut up the rest into pieces for us kids and put the food on our individual plates, which you bring to our cozy six-person table by the window, placing each one beside our little cups of milk or water. Your small frame moves quickly, purposefully.

Brother, I can hear you in the backyard as you kick a soccer ball around. You are perpetually playing sports. You are tall, lanky, and athletic, and all my friends think you are cute. We are only a year apart, but because you are a boy and I am a girl, we have different interests. You like to play video games and watch TV. I like to play with dolls and read. But we are usually not very far away from each other. We are like a team of two, the way my girls will be 30 years later. Sometimes, you barge into my room to ask if I want to play tennis in the street or watch TV with you. "Maybe later," I say.

Sister, you live in the room next door, pulling toys from the shelves and making a huge mess on the floor. You are a spunky five-year-old blond with bright blue eyes and a gregarious personality that is in stark contrast to my shy demeanor. Without even seeing you, I know you are dressed up in some sort of costume with a hat and maybe some make-up. "Just stay out of my room," I think. You are always running clumsily and loudly around the house. "Be careful," I yell through the wall. "You don't want to get stitches again!" It was just a few years ago that you slammed yourself into the corner of a dresser and had to have more than 30 stitches on your mouth. We are on high alert around you, but you keep us laughing.

Little Brother, I am obsessed with you. With your pudgy cheeks and big green eyes, you are so adorable that I treat you like you are my baby, which I know annoys you. You play quietly with your cars and figures, probably lining them up in some complicated configuration, pausing only to ask Mom when dinner will be ready or asking what the rest of us kids are doing. I have all sorts of baby names for you even though you are already four years old.

"Dinner!" Mom would scream. You yell it at least five times before all of us make it to the table. Dad, you arrive like clockwork as soon as we sit down. 6pm on the dot. You take off your hat and coat, put down your briefcase, and come straight to the kitchen. No need to decompress. You are hungry and excited to sit down with the family. Your suit and tie are still in place, and your hair is combed neatly to the side. Behind your glasses, you seem to be thinking. I know you could outsmart almost anyone, but with us you are caring and sweet.

The meal goes fast – boisterous and messy and filled with life. We talk about our days, we fight, we laugh and make fun of each other. The food doesn't have much taste, but it doesn't matter. When we finish, Dad you will help Mom clean the kitchen and we kids will head to their bedroom to watch some TV before bed. Mom and Dad, you will continue to catch up after we fall asleep. When the door is closed, it is your time together. I never hear you two fight.

On the weekends, we pile into the grey minivan and take trips, the little ones on the middle bench, me and the older brother in the back. Sometimes we go to the beach, carrying sandwiches in a bag and umbrellas, towels, and chairs under our arms. Sometimes we head to a historic site or garden. We always stop at a fast-food joint on the way back. I can remember exactly what everyone liked to order at Nathan's or Wendy's. I can hear us singing songs and telling jokes. I can picture the faded grey texture of the seats. When we get home, we curl up in our beds and fall asleep.

Every day was the same. So much stability, so much support, so much love. It was like we lived in a bubble. It would stretch one way, move a little another way, lose a bit of air, and then grow bigger. It was constantly there protecting me. I trusted it so much that I didn't even see it. It never crossed my mind that it could pop.

Not much changed in those years, except that we got older. Soon I am reading Catcher in the Rye and staring at the ceiling of my bedroom with my boyfriend. My brother begins to rebel against my parents, but we remain friends. I grow embarrassed by my sister's eccentricities but remain secretly flattered that she follows me around. My little brother is still the baby, trying to find his own way.

Mom, you would hire babysitters and cleaning ladies, and sometimes find a job outside of the house, but mostly it is you holding us together at home. Dad, you commute to the city every day and will continue to do so for more than 20 years. Every morning you wake at 6:11am and chug a glass of orange juice and then a glass of milk to get you started.

The weekend minivan trips continue even after my brother and I grow embarrassed to be seen with the family. I remember that feeling of piling into the minivan so well, the slight smell of mildew, the shrieks of my siblings, the large windows to the outside. To Adventure Land, the diner, Colonial Williamsburg, the Catskills, skiing, and the arcade. My friends make fun of the minivan and, I will admit, I grow slightly embarrassed. "Your family is so big!" they would say. "You are always together."

Then one day I graduated from high school and packed up my things for college. I am excited to be on my own. Brother, you visit me occasionally, and we stay good friends. I have less and less in common with our little siblings, who are in middle school now, but we talked on the phone anyway. Mom and Dad, you call every day, but I learn quickly that I don't have to tell you everything, and our relationship starts to change. I am growing up.

Yet I know that no matter what roads I crossed, we will always have one another and our memories of a life that, despite feeling boring at times, is perfect in retrospect.

Looking back, it was the reliable bubble that we shared that I could always go back into if I felt like it. As I grew up and started to experience life's hardships, all I wanted was to go back there, inside that bubble, with you guys.

Mom and Dad, you finally sold the house in Long Island. I didn't think you would go through with it. I had been trying to convince you to move for years. The neighborhood had changed and the layout of the house no longer suited your lifestyle. Much to your disappointment, it was seldom that we all gathered there like old times.

I went for our final family dinner at the house, and, while my girls played, I lingered in my old bedroom packing up memorabilia: the art on the wall, the box of Barbie dolls and doll clothing, the stacks and stacks of paperback books, the varsity swim jacket and Bat Mitzvah dress still hanging in the closet, the bag of love letters from my high school boyfriend tucked aside nearby. I laughed as I surveyed the room for the last time. My childhood has been emotionally gone for decades, but we were finally leaving it physically behind. You kept it for as long as possible. I reminisced about growing up there and how much I would miss it – that world, that bubble – now that the bubble has burst.

Sincerely,
Shanna

Dear Grandma,

Sometimes I still get the urge to pick up the phone and call you. "Shanna?" you would say. "How are you? Tell me something!" I can hear your voice like it was yesterday, even though it has been years since you died.

I loved our conversations. I would blab on about my friends, my schoolwork, and later, my job, my life in the city, my new life in the suburbs, my husband and the kids. "Are you eating well?" you would ask. "Are you happy?" Then you would end with, "Thank you so much for calling. You made my day. I love you so much. You are a doll. When are you coming for a visit?"

When I was younger, at least once a year, sometimes twice, we would head south. We would take the Amtrak auto train, where our car was put on the train and we sat and slept upfront in train seats. Other times, we would drive all the way down to Florida, all of us jammed into the minivan for 25 hours stopping overnight in some shady roadside motel. When we arrived, it was like we had made it to the promised land. You welcomed us with open arms, coming down to the parking lot with kisses and hugs to help us with our luggage. Inside your apartment there would be a giant spread of all the foods you knew we loved: marble cake, tuna mixed with relish, soft alpine Swiss cheese, bagels, chopped liver. We would eat for over an hour, and you would say, "Did you have enough? Let me cut up some fruit." Then we would go to the pool and relax on the lounges, our skin growing brown. At night, the kids shared the rickety pullout couches in your small living room. My parents slept in your room, and you slept in your friend's apartment downstairs.

Once in high school, I brought my boyfriend with us. In college, I brought my freshman-year girlfriends, and then my senior-year girlfriends. When my husband and I starting dating, he came down, and soon our children joined us. I wonder what you thought of these people who came into my life – and then into yours. You welcomed them all.

At night, we would plan an activity together. We'd go to the horse track, or the movies, or the mall; we'd go to one of your favorite restaurants. Even as my siblings and I grew up, the routine didn't change. You never seemed to lose any energy or look any older.

Thankfully, you lived a long and healthy life. Not an easy one, though. Your family didn't have a lot of money. You grew up in a time when women were supposed to be homemakers – and you were good at being a wife and mother. But you were smart and articulate, and I wonder if you were fulfilled. When you were a young woman, you lost one of your brothers on D-Day during World War II. You lost your husband, my grandfather, suddenly to a heart attack when he was only in his 50s, and then your second husband two decades later to cancer. You lived far away from your children and grandchildren, and you got lonely.

But none of that suffering showed. You were always positive and energetic, with a twinkle in your eye, a huge toothy grin and a boisterous laugh. I knew about everything you had endured, and I couldn't believe you got through it all without losing your wit and optimism. You were a guidepost and a source of comfort and strength for everyone around you.

There you are in my mind's eye with your blond hair sprayed to perfection, your red lipstick and mascara, in some brightly colored striped outfit. And all that costume jewelry. I used to play with it when I was younger: the pinky ring with the hanging gold coin, the chunky necklaces and bracelets and pins that coordinated with whatever you were wearing. You were always so put together. Your eyes were big and blue, your voice low, clear, and a bit raspy.

Let's be honest – you could have had any guy in the apartment complex. Men clamored after you. After your husbands died, you "dated" a man who was like another grandfather to us. He had a permanent seat on the chair in front of your TV.

And you had an entourage. Your best friends often accompanied us on our family night outings. They would tell us about the olden days in New York and what their grandchildren were doing. You would be on and off the phone with them, gossiping for hours. You loved to have people around you.

I idealized the relationship you had with my mom. Every time the phone rang at her house, I knew it was you. Reporting on the weather in Florida, a funny story you wanted to share, your last errand, what you planned to do with the rest of your day. In return, my mom told you everything that was happening in her life: what she was making for dinner, the latest with the kids, drama with her friends. I thought it was sweet that you shared everything with each other, sometimes multiple times a day. Always a good morning call. Always a goodnight call.

Like you, my mom wants to know everything that is going on with me. "How was your day?" she asks. What happened at work, class, school, with the kids, over the weekend? First in phone calls, now with texts. I do not enjoy sitting on the phone reviewing the day, analyzing people and places and events. I prefer to spend my time living my life and exploring new things. And relaxing and digesting it by myself. I guess I am more of an introvert. I don't want to share my every move, my every thought. You understood me. My mom understands me too.

You died in the middle of my chemo regimen for the Stage 2 diagnosis. I felt awful that winter; it was an out-of-body experience, a true roller coaster experience. "Who is this?" I would think as I faced the skinny, pale, sick, bald person in the mirror. My parents moved in and lived with me for six months. My mom fed me every meal, helped me walk around the house, rubbed my feet while I napped. She played with my girls. She gave me positive thoughts to help heal my grieving heart. I needed her. At night, she would retreat to our guest room and call you to recount the day—the doctors' appointments, how I looked, how I felt. I spoke to you only once or twice during that period. "How are you, darling?" you asked.

"Not good,"

"Shanna, don't worry. You are going to be fine," you told me in your sunny, confident voice. I wanted to believe you.

And then one rainy week in March, you called my mom to say you didn't feel well and were going to the hospital. I told my mom to go to Florida. Two days later, you were gone. My mom cleaned out your house and was back by the end of the week. Back to nursing me, helping me with household tasks, with the kids.

I feel guilty that my illness happened during the final months of your life. Did your suffering become too great watching your young granddaughter fight a terrible disease? Did you decide to leave when Mom was distracted with me? Or was the timing a coincidence?

I did not think my mother would get over your passing. Afterwards, she berated herself for not seeing it coming, even though you were 93 years old. The hole in her world was gaping. How would she get through each day?

Grandma, what is my role with the women in my family now? Can I support my mom in the way she needs to be supported? Who will support my sister? Will my daughters and I talk the way you and Mom talked? I wish you were here so I could ask you.

Your final wish for me was that I help others. I hope that you can read this book from wherever you are and be proud of it.

Sincerely,
Shanna

Dear Younger Self,

Did you ever imagine that in your thirties you would have a life-threatening disease? Unbelievable, right? Unfathomable, I know. Well, guess what? All the experiences you are having now are preparing you for it. You are on a slow steady incline that will give you the strength you need to live, and even thrive, with the Big C.

The truth is that it will take you about 18 years to come out of your shell.

When you are young, you will be painfully timid. You will have a few friends at the Elementary and Middle School with whom you will play dolls and games quietly; sometimes you will have sleepovers and watch movies into the night. Yet that won't be good enough for you. You will observe the social dynamics around you, and you will want to be "louder," more "popular," and with more "fun" kids. But you won't have the confidence to make that happen. It will be easier for you to retreat and be with the friends you are most comfortable with. You will think maybe you aren't cool. You won't realize then that the other kids probably don't notice you. If you went up to them and asked them to play with you, they probably would!

How do I know this? Because I am a parent now to two beautiful girls. One of them, the oldest, was also shy as a young child. I noticed that when she was more outgoing, the other kids would play with her. I suggested she try it more, and I was right. Now she is the biggest social butterfly I know. When I dropped her off at sleep-away in July (the summer before 3rd grade), I tried to introduce her to the girls in the bunk beds next to her. She looked at me and said, "I already introduced myself, Mommy," and they ran off together.

I also know because eventually you will figure it out for yourself.

When you are in High School, there will be a girl on your swim team who is in the "cool" group. She will be nice to you and you will go out for lunch together almost every day. One day, on your walk to the pizza place, out of nowhere you will ask her if you can hang out with her and her friends on the weekend. She will look surprised but say, "Sure!" She will invite you to one of the girls' houses. The next thing you know, you will have a new group of friends. These girls will be so pretty and nice and fun. You will keep your old friends, who are mostly your study buddies in your honors classes, but you won't believe how easy it is to suddenly have a whole new outlet! The new girls will like you. You will chat on the phone for hours. You will drive to the boat docks on Saturday night to meet the boys, and sometimes go to clubs in the city. You will pay more attention to how you dress. You will slowly grow into yourself.

Sleep-away camp during the summers will also be a time of growth. You will go to sleep-away camp for seven consecutive summers, all the way through high school. Although you won't participate much in sports (except tennis), you will love the art activities and the social events. The boys will talk to you. You will learn to dance. You will have a group of friends who make you laugh. At times, they will be cliquey; sometimes you will be part of the clique and sometimes you will be on the outside. Sometimes they will call you spaced out or make fun of you. It will make you sad, but it will toughen you up.

This social awareness, this ability to connect with people – and deal with the tough ones – will help you manage your disease. You will need to develop strong relationships with your doctors. You will need to navigate very complicated situations and understand the people behind them to advocate for yourself. You will need support, and you will find that support in health service professionals, support groups, work colleagues, new friends, old friends, and family.

And you will have to go back to the core of what fulfills you and makes you happy every day.

The truth is that it will take you about 21 years to really figure out what that is.

You will get bored easily as a child. For better or worse, your family will stay to themselves. Your siblings will keep your parents busy, and you will long for more activities to do outside. You will become jealous when you see people going to BBQs and other social events. You will spend countless hours reading to pass the time. Listening to music. And doing your homework. You will be a straight-A type of kid.

You won't be very good at sports. And you will know that is a problem because the cooler kids are good at sports. You will never try to get better; you just won't play them. In gym class, you will be one of the last picked for the team. You aren't coordinated. And you are skinny, without much energy or muscle tone. When you run, you get cramps under your ribs. Your parents won't do much to help develop you athletically. Anyway, you aren't interested in sports.

You aren't sure what you are interested in. You like art. You like music. You like being quiet. But you also yearn for excitement, for energy. And you aren't sure where to find it.

You will have a boyfriend in high school. He will notice you and court you until you become serious for over two years. He will take you to concerts, and you will go to parties and dances. You will start to experience new things. You will continue the swim team. You will get involved in Model Congress and recognize that you have an interest in thinking through problems and debating them in public. For many sessions, you will sit listening to the kids debate each other and you will be jealous of their banter and intellect. You have ideas, too; you just can't get them out. Then one day, you will be put in a group where you don't know anyone. This is your chance, you will realize, because you don't care what they think of you. You will get up there and start to talk. Then you will get up again and again. Your arguments will be solid. Your confidence will grow stronger. Later that day, in front of the entire program, you will be awarded best speaker! You will never forget what it feels like when they announce your name and you walk up to the podium in front of what feels like a thousand people. Everyone will be clapping and the people you know will be yelling your name. You will blush but accept the medal with ease. When you bring it home that night, Dad (ever the lawyer) will be so proud of you. Together you will hang it up on the wall.

You will always like art but you won't take it seriously until high school. By then, you will have started to take the lead on anything artistic at camp, like painting color war team plaques. At school, you will have the choice to take electives and within a few years will have taken every art class offered. I still remember the pride you feel when people call you well-rounded and creative. You will be a good student, a social student, and a student who takes AP Art and is selected to draw and paint for special high school events. It will be you who illustrates the dance tickets and the inscription placed inside the library books.

In college, your artistic expression will escalate and you will work towards earning a Minor in Fine Arts. You will set up a studio in your apartment and paint and draw almost every week. It will become a way to express yourself and differentiate yourself.

Then you will become adventurous and decide to change it up completely. You will enroll in a study-abroad in Belgium. You think it will be an enriching opportunity, and, since you don't know anyone else who is going, a fresh start. You will be living in a small college town, which will be a break from the city of Philadelphia. And you will be able to travel and enjoy as much of Europe as possible. You will arrive early with a couple of friends and explore France and Italy. During the semester, you will make new friends and take a different trip each week: to the Netherlands, Denmark, Germany, Spain, and all around Belgium. Your mom will visit for a weekend, and you will go to London. You will realize that you love to travel. And to be friends with people from different backgrounds.

I bet you still remember what it was like to live in Belgium, with Belgians, Italians, Danes, Australians, and Americans from all over the country (some who grew up on farms, some who went to small schools, some who were from the West Coast). How you felt like you were in another universe – and another era, for that matter. How enchanting the churches and medieval buildings were. How delicious the mouth-watering frites and chocolates tasted. The sound of European techno music blasting in the pubs late into the night. The European fashion-forward styles in the boutiques. The accents of people who came from completely different backgrounds, the amused look on the shopkeepers' faces when you ordered food and drinks in your broken Flemish. The Euro-rail pass in your wallet that was getting worn from all the punches received from train conductors.

All these adventures, this soul-searching, this quest for self-knowledge will help you tremendously when you live with breast cancer. Many patients I know start looking desperately for what to do with their potentially "limited" time. What fulfills them? What makes them happy? For you, these questions will already have been answered. You will already have discovered that you want to create art, travel the world, and be with the people you hold close to you. You will also have learned that you like to dissect complicated issues and share with others (thus the writing of this book).

So, dear Younger Self, now you head up, up, up the roller coaster, to a future of highs and lows, and fortunately a lot of steady ground in between.

And one day in your thirties, you will face the biggest descent of your life.

You will also rise to the highest heights of your life.

You will be back to writing, painting, traveling, and all the activities that you love. It will feel so good to go back to your core – to ways of living that make you feel the most like yourself, the person you always were, even before you knew it.

I think about you all the time, about the journey you will take and the challenges you will face. Trust the process and know that one day it will all make sense.

Sincerely,
Shanna

Dear September 11th Victim,

Every year on September 11, I think about you. When the kids are at school and my husband is at work, I turn on the TV for the 9/11 ceremony and curl up on the couch in the quiet house. It is my private ritual of remembrance.

As soon as I hear the two bells signifying the moments when the towers were hit, I am transported into my 23-year-old self at the bottom of one of the craziest roller coaster ride of my young adult life. There I am at work, on the 42nd floor of the World Financial Center. Puzzled by a sudden and fierce crash, I ran to the window and looked up. In the building, right across from ours and about 20 floors up, I saw a gaping hole and people jumping out of it. They looked so little. Like little dolls. But yes, they were people. Men wearing suits and ties. They jumped and flipped over a few times in the air. One at a time.

An older colleague was standing next to me. "I have seen this before," he said. "People get stressed and jump to their deaths." I was confused. Weren't they jumping because of the gaping hole? Maybe he was right. He was a VP, after all. I went back to my cube. There weren't many people in the office. There was simultaneously a stillness and an energy in the air. I felt like I was dreaming.

A couple of people were walking down the hallway. One told me he heard that a helicopter had gone off track and hit one of the Twin Towers. I felt horrible, but also relieved that this probably wasn't going to affect me. Unfortunately, dear victim, it was going to affect you.

Soon an alarm went off and the speaker system announced that a plane had hit one of the Twin Towers and more information would be provided as it became available. I walked back to the window and saw that the hole had become bigger and fiery. The fire was growing quickly.

My heart rate was going up. I felt nauseous and hot. I was pacing in my cube. Why did I have to come to work early on this out of all days? I thought. Why did you, dear victim?

When the second plane hit the second Twin Tower, I felt our building shake and I knew I was in danger. One of my colleagues ran past my desk with her backpack on and a look of terror on her face.

I grabbed my purse and headed to find my Vice President, who was sitting at her desk. She looked calm. I had always been intimidated by her. After all she was older than I and two levels above me. My job was to please her. "I think we should go," I said, and we went together down the hallway.

At the stairwell, we found a crowd of people jammed into the very small space. The company's General Manager was in there instructing the employees to stay put. "Go to back to your desks, everyone," he said.

No one understood what was going on. No one knew what to do. Everybody was silent, but there was panic surrounding us. My VP and I pushed forward into the stairwell. Together, we walked down 42 flights of stairs, round and round. I held tightly to the railing. I lost sense of time. I was wearing black pants and a blue shirt. Black heels, no socks. My feet were killing me.

Towards the bottom, I saw daylight, and exhaled a huge breath. Outside there were fire trucks, policemen, alarm sounds everywhere. Huge crowds of people. Radios blaring. What I remember most was the smell. A putrid smell of fire mixed with chemicals. I looked up and the sky was filled with smoke: two huge clouds coming from the Twin Towers, churning and growing.

My VP and I found a couple of colleagues, and we walked together up the West Side Highway. One of them explained that there was a terrorist organization that had flown planes into the

Twin Towers in a pre-meditated attack. 'Suicide bombers' he called them. He told us that the Pentagon had also been hit. My VP remained calm. I was about to lose my shit. "It's good versus evil," our colleague said. I had no idea what he was talking about.

We were a small group amongst what it seemed like millions of people. The safe ones. I didn't realize at the time that I had already survived. You, dear victim, were still up there. Somewhere.

We continued walking in a single line up the Hudson River, covering our mouths with our sleeves. The smoke was everywhere, and my eyes were stinging. I remembered that my brother was working in the other World Financial Center. I pulled out my cell phone to call him but there was no reception.

At around Canal Street, we heard a growling crash. Like a volcano erupting. We spun around. One of the Twin Towers was collapsing. It looked like it was melting. In seconds, we saw it crumble to the ground, and it was gone. Were you in that Tower? I still can't fathom that thousands of people like you perished in just the amount of time it took to turn my eyes and blink my eyes. What did it feel like?

"Where should I take you?" my VP asked.

"My mom works in Union Square," I said. "You can take me there."

Approaching 14th Street we heard another crash. This time we knew exactly what it was. We turned around. The other Twin Tower was gone.

My mom was working as an assistant at an architectural firm. In her office, we found her colleagues huddled in a conference room watching the television and the scene I had just been part of. "Mom," I said and went over to her. She had an unfamiliar glassy look in her eyes. I thought she would have screamed and hugged me, but she was eerily quiet. Like she was in a trance. My VP left, and my mom and I walked to my apartment nearby. We turned on the TV. When my roommate came home, we made pasta. The cell phones still didn't work.

Later that night we reached my brother, who was home safely on the Upper East Side. We called my dad and decided that my mom would stay with me. I called my boyfriend, now my husband, who was in California on a business trip. He had been trying to call me and was unable to get through to me all day. I told him I was safe.

During the next week, my college friends gathered in one another's apartments. None of us were going to work and none of us were going the next week either. We had nothing to do. That weekend we went to our Fire Island share house. It felt different from the other party weekends we'd shared over the summer. It was somber and quiet. There was hardly anyone else on the island. We cooked meals and sat on the deck. Time stood still.

For weeks, my roommate and I walked over to the memorial at Union Square, a sea of pictures of the missing, candles, flowers, music. Every day, it grew bigger and bigger. I cried so hard that my body shook. I imagined my own picture and name in the New York Times *Lost Persons* section. Missing: 23 years old, analyst at a large corporation. Last seen on the 42nd floor. Was there an ad made for you? How old were you? Where did you work?

I spoke to friends and heard more stories. My colleague's friend had perished into thin air. A father in my home town was gone. My friend's friend from college had survived after walking down 101 flights in the second Twin Tower. Did you have a chance of surviving? Did you make it to the stairwell? I never turned off the TV. The death toll grew.

My office building was badly damaged. The glass ceiling had imploded into the Winter Garden, where we had celebrated our Christmas party with overflowing platters of martinis and lobsters and a 12-piece band. The glass siding of the World Financial Center had shattered, office furniture and papers strewn all over the place.

Putrid smells filled the hallways. The fiery holes continued to burn next door with smoke clouds floating through the city and across to Brooklyn and New Jersey. Your office building was gone.

We were relocated to New Jersey. It was a strange time. We sat in bumper-to-bumper traffic on buses and in cars to get to and from work. Some people seemed to be able to move on; others could not. Grief counselors came to the office. Colleagues cried inconsolably in their cubicles.

Earnings were reported and it was announced that the company was struggling financially. Thousands of layoffs were made. Colleagues who were still in shock and grieving were told they no longer had a job. I watched as they packed up their belongings and left. I was "lucky" to keep my job, but I felt flat and empty inside. I didn't even know you but I was grieving for you.

Eight months later we were transferred back to our old building, with a view of the still-burning holes in the ground next door. The furniture and carpets were brand new. There was a shiny silver picture frame on each of our desks from the CEO to welcome us back. Our company was one of the first to come back to the area. Downtown was now a ghost town. Blockades on every street. It took almost 30 minutes to get to the subway that used to be across the street.

Consultants were hired and reports were published. Don't worry, they said. It is safe to be here. But it didn't feel safe. It felt too soon. It felt wrong. There was nothing I could do about it except hold my breath when I was next to the fiery hole. And when I was going up to the now 43rd floor on the elevator.

I was working in a new group now, with a new job internally, and we focused on getting the job done. But it was a long transition back to normalcy, which pretty much spanned my 20s.

My boyfriend traveled a lot for his job, and when he left I would cry uncontrollably, certain that something bad was going to happen to him. We started taking vacations again, but I was terrified of flying, sure the plane was going to crash into something. He held my hand tightly as my heart beat out of my chest.

In hindsight, I realize I should have been working with a professional. I was experiencing intense anxiety. My hair was falling out in clumps. I had a few visits to the ER after my heart raced so fast I feared I was having a heart attack. They sent me home each time and told me it was stress. I would weep walking down the street. Weep sitting in my apartment. I thought I had cancer. I went to doctor's appointments and begged them to check my skin one more time, test my blood one more time. "You are fine," they always said. But I never felt fine.

Eventually the city started to recover, and so did I. The restaurants once again filled with people. The real estate market climbed. Business started to grow. My boyfriend and I got engaged and moved in together. We got married, went on our honeymoon. I got promoted and my husband's job as a financial analyst began to take off. My girls were born. We moved to the suburbs.

But I never went to work again on September 11th or did much of anything on that day. My husband does; sometimes he even flies on business trips. Every year I sit in my home and am brought right back to that day that changed me forever.

Now I see my life as divided into pre-September 11th and post-September 11th. The day I saw the world for what it really was: a frightening, unpredictable, uncontrollable place. But it was also the day I saw people being their authentic selves, motivated not by money and power, but by their humanity and their willingness to help others.

A decade after the tragedy, I started noticing headlines connecting cancer and 9/11. At first, they talked about the first responders – the firemen who ran into the building, the workers who cleaned up the fiery remains. They got lung cancer and mesothelioma. They were on disability. They were dying. Then it was about more than that. There was a report that referenced thousands of people who lived and worked in the area getting cancer. Breast cancer, ovarian cancer, skin cancer, brain cancer. All kinds of cancer. All kinds of people. I didn't pay too much attention. I didn't have cancer.

And then I did. After I was diagnosed with breast cancer in November 2012, I wondered about 9/11. Was it the cause of my disease? The fumes, the sooty smoke, the endless terror. It made perfect sense to me. I had feared cancer for so long. And on 9/11, I thought I was going to die. So, I wasn't crazy: September 11th was killing me. I had known all along.

Dear victim, you haunt me every year. You died and I lived. But for how much longer? Your fate frightens me. But why? It will be mine one day, too. Only time is what separates us on this crazy roller coaster ride.

Sincerely,
Shanna

Dear Husband,

When people ask how we got together, you always tell the whole long story. I think it's so cute and endearing, because, frankly, I just say, "We met in college."

But you tell anyone who asks all the details. The facts, the coincidences, the irony of it all. Another one of life's roller coasters.

The day we were introduced I was 17 and a senior in high school, visiting the College with my friend to see if we liked it. You were a freshman. We stayed with my friend from home who was also your fraternity brother. After a night of heavy drinking with your friends, my friend and I sat opposite you at a pizzeria on 41st Street in West Philadelphia for a recovery brunch. You tell people that I was wearing my glasses and pajamas. And that you couldn't stop staring. I also noticed your intense brown eyes right away and the narrow face. Some freckles scattered across the bridge of your nose and your fair complexion. Your wavy hair. And your approachable and confident way.

For the three years that we overlapped in College, our paths kept crossing. We passed on the college walk in front of the library, with our books on our backs and our friends flanking us. My girlfriends and I appeared at your fraternity parties in packs of black pants, long hair, and made-up faces (although I was the one not wearing any!). One year, we dressed as "skaters" for your annual Halloween party, wearing ski hats and baggy jeans and holding skateboards. My girlfriends and I danced for a while before deciding it was time to go to the next fraternity party. You were watching us from the side of the room, with your friends who were visiting from Montreal. I had no idea.

Throughout college, I thought you were nice and friendly. Always said hello and would strike up a conversation. Different from other guys, who were hard to differentiate from the rest of their fraternity. I thought it was cool that you were from Montreal. And that your name was different. What an interesting name. I heard that your dad was an orthodox rabbi and that you were somewhat of a rebel. I liked you. But I never thought there was anything beyond that.

One day my parents called me and told me they had met the parents of a guy with your name who went to my college. They were all sitting at the pool in the town in Florida, where my grandma lived. And your grandma lived. Your mom and my dad also realized they were both from Brooklyn. We had the same type of upbringing. Similar roots. A sign.

I continued to see you at parties or on campus. You were always popping up. It was like we were in similar social scenes but different actual circles. I remember calling you for some tips when my friends and I decided to go to Montreal for spring break.

I had a series of monogamous relationships through college. Apparently, you asked me out a couple of times, and I made some bad excuses. I don't remember that. Or why I made excuses. I think I knew you liked me. But I was focused on other things. Like chasing guys who probably didn't like me.

After I graduated, I bumped into you on the Long Island Rail Road. You were by yourself on your way to visit your brother, who, it turned out, lived in the same town I'd grown up in. We chatted about the suburbs and what it was like to live in the city post college. I was still wearing my pajamas. I liked to be comfortable but you kept catching me wearing them. Another sign.

I had just started working in Lower Manhattan. One day I met my mom for lunch downstairs from my office. There you were again. This time, all cleaned up and in a suit. Ordering your lunch right in front of me on line. We exchanged business cards. I introduced you to my mom. "Cute," she whispered in my ear.

That afternoon I called you. I'm not sure why. I think I knew that you weren't going to call me. And that the ball was in my court if I wanted to see you again. So technically our relationship started because I asked you out. To a concert that night. You love to tell people that detail.

After that, we were together. On the roller coaster. Until then, it was like we were drifting around with the universe trying to get us to stick, and it was only a matter of time until that happened. We dated for three years before you proposed. Bouncing around from my apartment on the Upper East Side and then Union Square, to yours in SoHo and then the East Village. Eating out. Traveling. Going to parties. Introducing each other to our large circles of friends and family. Most of all, we had fun. Although personality-wise we couldn't be more different (you are loud and in the moment; I am shyer and more thoughtful), we balanced each other out. You have always felt like home to me.

From the day we met, until we got married, it was almost 10 years. Our wedding was at a temple in Long Island, a couple of miles from my parents' house. One topic we discussed at length was how much religion would be involved. Neither of us had any problem voicing our opinions, and I remember having fights that would last hours. Both of us screaming at each other. I read that when you fight that early in a relationship, it is not a good sign. I knew in my heart we had issues to work out. And that is what we did.

We set up a wedding registry. We started a bank account together with our wedding money. We bought furniture, took out a mortgage, and did all the other adult things you are supposed to do. We built our foundation together. We have lived in three apartments and two houses. We have traveled the world. We have been to hundreds of restaurants. We have had our children and settled down. Now we have been married for 15 years.

Looking back, I see how young and naïve we were. Our life felt intense sometimes, but we were blessed with stability for many years. Yes, there were ups and downs: September 11th. Trying to get pregnant. Your various job searches. Searching for a house. Weathering the post-2008 economic recession. Your career in the hedge fund business. Thousands of hours of business travel and working around the clock. Your dad's stroke.

But it wasn't until my diagnosis that our real journey began. And we would do it together, in love and in partnership.

Sincerely,
Shanna

Dear Girls,

I remember when each of you were born. Your personalities were front and center right from the start.

To my eldest: when they put you on my chest, I stared into your big, deep-set brown eyes. I felt like I could gaze into your soul. You had the biggest cheeks I have ever seen and the cutest curls. A little button nose, like me. You were fiercely independent; shy at first, but eventually very social. When you started talking – way before anyone expected – you were so articulate: a smart, determined, sweet, and mature girl. You were always dancing and singing and are so graceful and beautiful. Quietly confident and so sure of yourself.

To my youngest: when you were born, you lay on my chest crying for over an hour. You were rattled and needed me to calm you down. I loved looking at your eyebrows, which match my own. And holding you. You are sensitive, compassionate and emotional, but somehow strong as a rock. Unique, cool and confident. A natural at pretty much everything, especially sports. You know so much and you learn everything by yourself. No shyness or holding back. Your uniqueness and talent is there for the world to see and admire.

Becoming a parent was not easy for me. In fact, it was my first personal struggle in life, and a roller coaster in and of itself. The first time I didn't get to plan exactly what I wanted. The first time I felt out of control.

For over a year, I had "unexplained" infertility. Daddy and I went from doctor to doctor and they told me to "just relax." After all, I was a healthy woman in my late 20s. It would happen in due time. But after six months of trying to no avail, we went to a fertility center on the Upper East Side, the one where everyone gets pregnant. We met the famous doctor, a short and boisterous

Mexican Jew, who gave me one look and said, "Don't worry, my dear. We will get you pregnant!"

I took Clomid for a few months before getting inseminated in their office at the perfect time of my cycle. When that didn't work, they suggested that I take injectable shots and then get inseminated, so there would be a higher chance of becoming pregnant. Every night I gave myself the shots in the bathroom. Every day I went in for blood work. Every month I was still not pregnant, and I cried my eyes out. I was bloated and uncomfortable. All my friends were pregnant or already had a baby. What was wrong with me?

We started the second cycle of injectable shots with a plan to move to IVF if it didn't work. We had been trying to get pregnant for a year and a half. I had lost over 10 pounds from the stress. I lied to almost everyone, including my parents, when they asked when we were having kids. I told them we weren't ready. Daddy was hopeful but I was miserable. I was sad and irritable and kept to myself.

That last cycle was during the summer. After the insemination, we went out for dinner in the city. We sat outside on the sidewalk. After not drinking for almost a year, I decided to have a couple of beers. Screw this, I thought. I drank again a week later at a concert in Williamsburg. And then one day, I woke up and realized that I was late. After tracking the days and minutes for so long, I had suddenly lost track of time. I looked at a calendar. I really was late!

The phone rang and it was a nurse from the fertility center. It was part of the protocol for her to check in. Until then, I had called her when I got my period, and we'd plan to start the next cycle. "When are you coming in for your pregnancy test?" she asked.

I was in denial. I took a pregnancy test at home first, and it was positive. I stared at that little line so closely that my vision doubled. I was in complete disbelief. How could this be? I had convinced myself that it was never going to happen. I had convinced myself that there was something wrong with me. I had convinced myself that I was going to be miserable forever. I was missing out on being a mom. And then, in an instant, the hell was over, and I saw my reflection smiling in the mirror. I called Daddy at work to tell him the good news. The next morning, we went to the clinic, and it was confirmed. We were going to have a baby. We were going to have a baby!

For the first three months, I continued to go to the doctor. They measured my blood levels and did weekly sonograms. We saw you in the blurry screen – a tiny speck in a world of blackness. Moving. Growing. After a couple of weeks, they found your heartbeat. It was so loud and fast and steady. I still couldn't believe it.

One day I went to find the doctor in the hallway to thank him and give him a bottle of wine. He gave me a high-five.

Then I transferred to the OB who delivered you, my first. I was so nervous. I kept thinking something would go wrong. But it was a perfect pregnancy. My belly grew bigger. You met all your milestones, as you always do. I felt you moving. I loved the way it felt at night; I would cuddle up with you and fall asleep. Daddy and I started to talk about furniture for the second bedroom and what to name you.

After you were born, I hired a baby nurse to help us for 10 days. She taught us how to swaddle you, bathe you, dress you, feed and burp you. Grandma and Grandpa, Tata and Saba, came over to spend time with you.

You were a small sweet angel. I loved dressing you up in the millions of outfits we had gotten for gifts. I would take you on long walks with new friends and their new babies. We had a routine. Me and you. You never worried me or gave me trouble. We were best friends from the beginning.

When I went back to work, I was conflicted. I took as long a maternity leave as possible. That first day I dropped you off at the daycare, I cried my eyes out. I knew I wasn't the type who could be a stay-at-home mom forever, and that you were going to benefit from daycare. But it still felt so hard.

After your first birthday, we started thinking about giving you a sibling. Knowing how long it had taken to get pregnant the first time, we started right away. And BAM, without any help, I was pregnant by August. We had planned a trip to Hawaii, and we went. When we came home, I went to the OB and she confirmed my pregnancy and found your heartbeat, little one. It was all happening so quickly. How were we this lucky?

After that we lived in the city, the four of us, for another 17 months. You girls shared a room. The carpet was the one we got from Turkey on our honeymoon. The colors on the walls and bedding were soft pink and green. The rocking chair was beige in a soft velvet.

The older one got a big bed, the little one got the crib. I had another maternity leave, and this time it seemed to go faster. Little one, you started daycare soon after. You were walking before you were 1. You were never far behind your sister. The two of you did everything together.

There is one day that sticks in my mind. It was a summer Tuesday, and it was movie night in our apartment complex. I rushed out of work and took the bus to the corner of 23rd Street and the FDR Drive. Then I walked west on 23rd and ran into the entrance of the daycare. I always had to put my purse through their metal detector. I said hello to the security guards and rounded the corner to that adorable center. I opened the door and said hello to the director. She was the mom of one of the little girls in the program. I unfolded the double stroller in the stroller room and wheeled it inside to pick up the two of you from your room. You both grinned and squealed when you saw my face. I shoved your bottles, extra clothes, and artwork into the bottom of the stroller. You had your usual bicker about who would sit in front, and that day the elder won. We headed out with more friends, chatting about our days.

Down the ramp and across the street to our apartment complex, our haven. Surrounded by dozens of red brick nondescript buildings. Past the mini tennis courts. Through the playground, lined with trees and filled with kids playing. Past the basketball courts. The air was warm but not too humid. We crossed the street and stopped at the deli to pick up some sandwiches and drinks, then continued into the development into the central circle. The fountain was on full force; it almost glowed. We stopped and you looked inside, studying the water with awe. I let you out of the stroller so you could run around. We waved when we spotted a couple of our neighbors. Then we kept going to the center of the circle where the movie was being projected. Hundreds of families were congregating. I pulled out the pink and brown blanket from under the stroller and spread out our food, including baby jars and a bottle for the little one. The movie was starting. It was my favorite – *Mary Poppins*! I saw Daddy running up behind us. He lifted you into the air one at a time, and your smiles were endless. We stayed for about half of the movie, until you both started falling asleep. Then we strolled home, you, little one, clutching your "night-night" and, you, the big one, sucking ferociously on your "paci." We brushed your teeth, changed your diapers, and got you into your PJs, and off to sleep you went.

Those years were like a slice of heaven. Yes, we had work and bills and stress, but they were in the background. In the foreground were the two of you. Gorgeous and precious babies. Growing every day. Swinging on the swings and running in the playground. Learning new words and making new expressions. Coloring and singing. Watching Disney shows. You were the light of both of our lives. We rushed home from work to see you and snuggle you.

Sincerely,
Shanna

November 21, 2012

Dear Cancer,

Today I was diagnosed with you.

Wait, did I just say that? Could it be? It seems impossible, but expected at the same time. I have been dreading – and waiting for – this day my entire life. The day you would get me.

When I was young, I had a strange suspicion that was I was going to die of cancer. I didn't know when or why, but I was certain it was going to happen. Every time I heard of someone being diagnosed with or dying from the disease, I paid careful attention to the story so when it happened to me, I would be prepared.

In high school my friend's mom died of ovarian cancer. One of my friends in college lost both of his parents to cancer. In 2005, my sister-in-law was diagnosed with metastatic melanoma and then with breast cancer a few years later. In 2010, my very dear friend was diagnosed with a serious form of blood cancer. The lightening kept striking, and it felt like you were getting closer and closer to me.

On November 21, 2012, out of the clear blue sky, I was diagnosed with Stage 2 breast cancer. I remember meeting with the oncologist in December after my double mastectomy to review the next steps. She looked calm, even bright-eyed. Her hair was dark brown and curly. She had probably already seen 10 other people like me that day. She told me to call her by her first name.

"The cancer is gone," she said. "You had clean margins. We got this, Shanna." I would have eight rounds of chemotherapy, some radiation to the chest wall, and then Tamoxifen for five years, a sort of insurance policy against any stray cells. "You are going to be okay," she said.

I wasn't reassured. Here I was, a 34-year-old mother of two amazing daughters, ages 1 and 3. And I have *cancer*. I have so much to live for, and you kill.

Plus, I knew I was going to lose my hair. I knew I was going to be sick as a dog. I was already 10 pounds thinner since the diagnosis.

I can see myself wearing my green button-down pajamas in her office. It was 8pm at night. My parents and my husband were sitting in chairs facing her. I was pacing around the room. I didn't believe I was going to be fine.

Suddenly I was nauseous. I felt the room go black, and everyone became blurry. I felt weight on my shoulders and I couldn't take a deep breath. I started crying and screaming, "I am going to die! I am going to die! I am going to die!"

"You are being treated, Shanna, but I'd better put you on some antidepressants," she said, and she hastily took out her prescription pad.

Two weeks later she called while I was driving. I had just started chemo and had a lot of concerns. I pulled into a parking lot, got out of my car, and started pacing by the grocery store's entrance. We went through my litany of questions: how to ease my constipation, how to manage the steroids, how to deal with my hair falling out. It was so casual. Like we were talking about the weather.

Then I asked, "What are the chances that after all this treatment, it will come back to another part of my body and kill me?"

She didn't miss a beat. "Around 30 percent," she said.

"And then what?"

"Well, you could have two more years. Maybe five, even 10."

The world went black again. I was falling fast down one of the sharpest descents of my roller coaster. The shoppers in the parking lot moved like fuzzy blobs in slow motion. The nausea came, and

I tried to take a breath but couldn't get any air. "I am going to die! I am going to die! I am going to die!"' I gasped.

"Shanna, listen to me. You will be cured," she said. "But I'd better change your antidepressant."

Did anyone out there realize how serious this was? You have a reputation of being curable. You have a reputation of being transient. You are not! We are not there yet! I hate you!

Sincerely,
Shanna

June 2017

Dear Body,

Nice job. You've hung in there, somehow. Past your median statistical expiration date of two-and-a-half years for a metastatic patient. Let's keep it going.

It hasn't been easy, I know. Every morning you are jarred awake by that nagging alarm that won't stop trying to get you out of bed hours before you are ready, even though you have slept for nine hours straight. From your warm and cozy cocoon, you pull yourself up after multiple snoozes. Throw on those comfy grey sweatpants and slippers and launch into your mommy duties: packing lunches, dressing and feeding the girls, driving them to school or camp, with a large cup of steaming caffeinated green tea as fuel. A couple slices of bread with peanut butter. Multigrain Cheerios with fruit if it's hot outside; steel-cut oatmeal with fruit if it's cold. And don't forget that handful of pills with a glass of water. Must take those damn chemo pills like clockwork, along with vitamin D for the bones, Prilosec for the acid reflux, probiotic for digestion, and Lexapro for anxiety.

After the kids are off, it's time to work out, sometimes at the gym and sometimes on the tennis courts. I try to do this at least three days a week, but you are often lethargic. The blood and oxygen feel like they have stopped flowing. It is a struggle to get you to move. But once I get your circulation going, I almost always feel better.

The first clue that the cancer had spread was when I hit the ball during a doubles tennis match. It was June 2014. I had been feeling frail and was still super skinny since the treatment for the Stage 2 cancer in 2013. Everyone was hopeful that I was in

37

remission, so I tried to be, too. But with that single swing of the racket, my life changed forever.

I felt a sharp, deep pull that started in my hip and gravitated up through my left glute, as if I had literally ripped something open inside of you. It was quick, but I knew I had never felt a sensation like that in all my life. "Ow," I said quietly, but the next game point was starting. We were close to the end of the match, and I played until we finished. How, I am not sure.

"Are you okay?" asked my partner as I limped off the court.

"I think so," I replied, but the area was sore and turning black and blue.

For the next two weeks I iced it, stretched it, massaged it, and rested it. I sat in Epsom salt baths. Twice I went to see the orthopedist, who told me that it was a classic injury and that I must have torn my glute. There was nothing to do but to wait for it to heal. I brought it up with the oncologist, but he wasn't concerned. I took Advil like clockwork, and the pain plateaued, but it was still there.

Nevertheless, my husband and I went to Peru for our 10th anniversary to explore Machu Picchu, the Sacred Valley, Cuzco, and Lima. We did a hike called Huayna Picchu, which is known as the "death hike" because of the steepness of the mountain. And we did it in the rain. On the way back, I slid and fell smack on my butt. A stab radiated through my lower back. I had probably made things worse, and it was stupid to have done the hike, but I kept wanting to believe that the pain wasn't there.

But you knew better, dear body. On the plane ride home, you spoke to me with such clarity that I knew that what I was experiencing was not just an injury. It was not nothing to worry about.

It was the cancer. In the bones.

On August 22, 2014, my husband and I waited all day for the phone call. We drove around in our car, through beautiful neighborhoods in Westchester, looking at the different styles of houses and gardens. We sat in the gazebo in the park watching the waves hit the rocks. Summer was turning into fall, and the air was getting cooler and crisper. The time went on and on.

I know, body, you felt like you were on speed. Like you wanted to run a marathon. But there was nothing to do but wait.

We were pulling into the house at 7pm when the phone rang. It was the oncologist. "It's cancer. It has spread to your bones." He said. "I am sorry."

It's odd that this time the world didn't turn black. Instead I felt separated from you, dear body. Like I was watching you receive the news. You did not cry. I did.

"What does this mean, doctor?" my husband asked, tears rolling down his face. I had seen him cry only a handful of times. We were sitting in the car on blue tooth speaker in front of the house talking into the air.

It meant that the disease had spread and was now incurable. It meant that there were drugs to treat it, but, as the oncologist said "you will live with it for the rest of your life. The cancer doesn't kill. People die when it causes problems in their organs."

"When will it happen? When will I die?" I asked.

"Only G_d knows," he answered.

I shook my head in shock. Here is the number one doctor in the world for breast cancer telling me that only G_d knows? I am in trouble.

After we hung up the phone, my two bodies merged back together, and I ran into the house and upstairs, avoiding my daughters and the babysitter in the family room. I called my parents to tell them, just like I had when I got into college, when I got engaged, when I got pregnant, when we bought a house and when I was diagnosed the first time. Hardly a tremor in my voice. "It's back", I said. "I knew it."

Then I hung up and fell onto my bed sobbing. Me sobbing when I found out the news is one of my daughters' first memories. They often talk about it. Remember when Mommy cried? Was it when you found out you had cancer? Yes, it was, my dears.

I was sad and crying but I noticed that my anxiety was gone. I had clarity for the first time in my life. It was all starting to make sense.

It was you I was worried about, dear body.

I pushed myself to heal you as quickly and efficiently as possible. After the radiation, I forged through a two-month physical therapy plan and then hired a trainer at the gym to work with me on a weekly basis. It has been years now, and I haven't missed a week.

That spring I joined the tennis team again, and that winter I joined an indoor racquet club so I could play tennis year-round. Then I added Thursday evening yoga to my schedule, with a spurt of hot yoga on the weekend. And long walks around the neighborhood.

Plus, the activity of being a young mom. Waterparks, trampoline parks, shopping sprees, carnivals, neighborhood picnics, bike rides – I have never missed out on an event. My family wants to do things, and so do I. When people whine about having too much going on and how tired they are, I quietly wonder whether, if they had Stage Four breast cancer, they would ever leave the house. Some days I don't think I can. But every day, I do it again. And again. And again.

Days turned into weeks. Weeks turned into months. Months turned into years. And here I am.

I am convinced that I can feel the cancer in my bones. My doctor is surprised, because most of the cells are in the marrow, which is impossible to feel. But I am sure I can. It's like fragile spots in parts of my skeleton. There is one on the back of my neck.

Another mid-spine. A large area on my lower back and sacrum (where the radiation was after the tennis injury ultimately revealed a spread to the bones). And then, in March 2017, in my left hip into the top of the femur.

My left femur is particularly weak; sometimes it seems like my leg is dragging when I walk or jog. I wonder if anyone can see it, but I know no one can. The sensation cycles up and down in intensity as the chemo pills work their way around my body. I am grateful that I have a marker to go by if there is further growth.

You have never failed me, dear body. Over and over, you adjust so I can go on with my routines. I know you don't like the treatments, as you have continually indicated with bouts of nausea, fatigue, diarrhea, redness and swelling. But with each medication, you ultimately absorb the toxicity and let the battle take place between the healthy cells and the sick cells.

What keeps you chugging along? Are the treatments helping you or hurting you? I believe the healing practices I have integrated – reiki, acupuncture, massage – have restored me. Plus, food, chocolate, sleep, music. You like these things, don't you?

When I was young, I thought I was weak. I was skinny and small-boned; not much muscle tone. Fertility treatments, pregnancy, and childbirth taught me that I was stronger than I knew. I created two babies!

But with the cancer, I am not sure.

You have made it through challenges that the toughest muscleman in the world might not have endured. I am proud of you. I am grateful to you.

Thank you, feet, for carrying me to the door of my house so I can go out.

Thank you, stomach, for putting up with the gruesome digestive side effects of my meds.

Thank you, skin, for tolerating all the creams and lotions necessary to keep the rashes away.

Thank you, brain, for letting me alleviate your chemical imbalances from all this trauma with anti-depression and anxiety meds.

Thank you, organs, for preventing the cancer from penetrating you (thus far).

Thank you, arms, for enabling me to cuddle my girls and husband at bedtime.

Thank you, hands, for allowing me to type these letters.

Please be good to me, dear body.

Please, let me see my girls grow.

Please, let me get on a plane and travel the world.

Please let me swim in the ocean, paint, dance and sing.

I promise I will be good. I will never second guess you.

Please show me the way.

Sincerely,
Shanna

Feel and Surround Yourself With Love

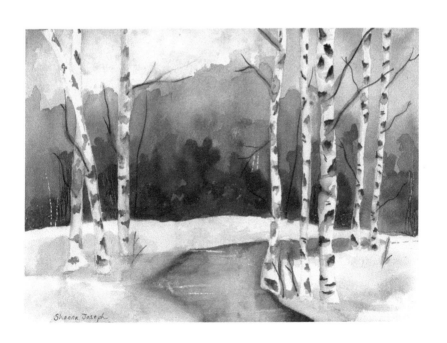

Shanna Joseph

December 31, 2013

Dear Higher Spirit,

Happy New Year.

What? Were you expecting me to thank you for letting me live? Sorry, but I am not feeling the least bit grateful. You've shaken me down to my core over the last year. There is almost nothing left of me. I am a dim light, flickering out, in a sea of darkness.

Just recently, I was shining brightly. A loving, supportive, successful husband: check. Two happy, beautiful daughters: check. A promotion to become one of the youngest VPs at my large corporation: check. A million-dollar-plus house in the suburbs, NY: check.

Good health: check.

I never thought much about you before. Never spent time praying to you or honoring you with appreciation. My accomplishments were the results of my own hard work and focus and had nothing to do with prayer or luck. You didn't like that, did you?

I guess you had to send me a severe message to get me to notice you. But did you have to wait until I had everything I had ever wanted before you knocked it all down? You can't have that, you said. You are not worthy. You do not deserve to be happy. I will destroy you.

Which you did. You traumatized me. You tortured me. You embarrassed me. And when I tried to get up, you kicked me down. To the lowest, scariest, and darkest place I could ever imagine. A place that made me want to disappear into the depths of the earth. Because I didn't care what happened to me anymore.

The day of my original Stage 2 diagnosis is etched clearly into my memory.

"You have cancer."

The tears falling down my husband's face. The doctor walking us through the hallway. The plan. My husband and I were shuttled from place to place, making decisions, setting dates. It was the longest day of my life. We walked together down the city blocks that we had moved from just months before and grabbed a slice of pizza for dinner.

Then it starts to blur. A year of hell, now reduced to snippets of sights, sounds, and sensations. The silence of the waiting room. Screams of pain. Complicated medical jargon. A medicine cabinet of pills. A river of tears.

I am on a table being wheeled into surgery, crying uncontrollably and shaking with terror. I am in the shower, trying to wash myself carefully around the drains and scars. I am sitting on a chair in a salon where a hairdresser is cutting my pony tail off in one swift motion. A bag of scarfs awaits at the bottom of my closet.

There I am, huddled into a chemo chair while a nurse pokes me again and again, trying to hook up the IV. She places a cup of pills next to a glass of water. Now I am giving myself daily shots in my bathroom before bedtime. A red cap covers my head so it doesn't get cold while I sleep. I see the image of my body in the mirror, scarred and getting thinner, paler, and balder.

Bottles of antidepressants. Uneaten meals. Waiting for another surgery. The hospitalization with doctors and nurses in masks and white plastic suits. Recovering on the couch. *American Idol. The Bachelorette.* Lying in bed. Lying on a chaise in my garden. Lying on a chaise at the pool.

The lights above me on the radiation table. The dressing gown. Stomachaches. Heartburn. Dry mouth. Dizziness.

The helpless looks on my parents' faces: my mom's sad, my dad's terrified. The sounds of the girls downstairs getting ready for school with the babysitter. The click of the door as they leave and I haven't said goodbye.

My spot in the corner of the couch again, where I lie too weak to reach for the remote control. This must not be my body.

The box of get-well cards. Many told me to have faith in you. That you would see me through this. I laughed bitterly when I saw those. What kind of idiots believe in G-d? I thought. If you do exist, you must really hate me.

My younger daughter doesn't want me. My oldest doesn't understand. My husband is running the house. I am useless. I am a ghost.

Why me?

I must have really needed a lesson.

I hate myself. I hate everyone around me.

Poor me.

This is a tunnel that goes on forever. No treatment will work. I am never going to get out of here. I am leaving my family. I am dying.

If my life were a stock, 2012 was the record high, 2013 the financial crisis. Except it didn't rebound. It is the Great Depression that never ends.

So, fine, I can see you now. You are trying to teach me a lesson. You scared the hell out of me and continue to scare the hell out of me. You may think that I should thank you for getting me through till now. But I cannot. You brought me to my knees. It is irreversible. I am a different person now. And for that, I will never forgive you.

Sincerely,
Shanna

January 1, 2014

Dear Husband,

Nothing could have prepared us for my diagnosis. It came out of the clear blue sky. I had a lump in my breast that was being 'checked' and 'biopsied.' This has happened before. The doctor was not worried. So much so that I went to the breast biopsy by myself, and you met me there on your way back from Barcelona. We thought it was annoying that the doctors were making me do this. I said I would see you after the procedure in the waiting room.

Then the doctor told me, "You have cancer." I realized they must have called you in. There was a five-second bit of time when I knew that our life was changing forever, but you didn't. I could tell by the sound of your footsteps in the hallway. They were light and steady. I heard you whistling. And then you came in, and I fell apart. I was crying hysterically. "I have cancer," I told you. "I'm going to die." I watched you process the news. Your expression changed from day to night. Two small tears rolled down your face. "No, you are not," you said. "We will figure this out."

That's you. Always the optimist. Always living in the present, not some imagined, terrifying future. You have been my rock through all of this. In the beginning you managed the appointments, the questions, the house, and the kids. As I became more comfortable with all the side effects and recovered from the mental stress, I took those on. But you remained my rock. Always the optimist. I don't think there is a more important role.

We keep going – traveling, doing activities with the girls, making plans for the house. I think if I ever see you falter, it will be the end of me. You keep me going on this roller coaster. Please don't stop.

Sincerely, Shanna

April 2014

Dear Girls,

You are my world. You are my heart. You are my purpose in life, the reason for my fight.

You are the extension of me. And ultimately you, and your kids, and their kids, will be my legacy.

How was it possible that it could change so drastically?

I look at pictures now from 2012 and it is unfathomable. There you are, playing by the fountain in the city. There you are, playing in the kitchen in our new house in the suburbs. And then there you are sitting next to me on the couch, and I am skinny and pale, and I am wearing a wig, with a blank look on my face. What I would give to freeze time and go back to those early days, those days before November 21, 2012. When the roller coaster began.

You and Daddy are the reason that I am even willing to take this ride.

Sincerely,
Shanna

August 2016

Dear Universe,

As my life moves in uncertain directions into uncharted territory, I have never felt more relaxed. Even, dare I say, graceful.

Don't get me wrong. I now live in a world filled with fear, uncertainty and outright terror. This is not visible to the human world. I will be at lunch with a friend, listening intently to her but also wondering how many lunches I will have left to enjoy with her. I will be at play with my kids, laughing and singing, but also wondering if I will live to see their adult selves.

But I can't deny that there has been a shift in the energy surrounding me.

For years, a little spirit sat on my shoulder, yelling in my ear, C'mon, make it happen: get an A, prove yourself, climb up the ladder, get in with the right people, move into a good neighborhood, make your family proud.

Now it is different. Gone are the days when I would shiver with anxiety – waiting for a boy to notice me, a group of friends to include me, a new boss to hire me, or, later promote me – wanting my life to move in a certain way. Gone are the more recent days when I would tremble with fear, waiting for a side effect to subside, or a doctor to tell me I was cured.

Now I float in mid-air. Now I fly from place to place, letting the wind carry me.

If I feel like taking a nap, I lay down. If I feel like taking a walk, I put on my sneakers. If I feel like seeing a friend, I call them and ask if I can come over.

It comes out in mundane ways, too. When I am driving, I am almost always listening to beautiful music now, instead of stressing about getting to my destination. When I am cooking,

49

I am enjoying the smells and the steps of creating, instead of stressing about getting dinner on the table at a certain time.

I have shifted from planning to living, from turmoil to peace, from terror to grace. With the support of my family, I have developed a spiritual practice that I believe sits at the core of my new existence. It started with visits to a reiki master and daily meditations. It has evolved to a new way of thinking, one rooted in exploration and being alive. I never did and probably never will believe in you, G-d (note though the holy and respectful spelling of your name and how it will always be spelled to me). But I have learned to let go, to surrender, to be okay with a life in which I have no control. And this is a place of acceptance and love.

Last weekend, my husband watched my daughters while my friend and I went on a retreat in the Berkshires. I'd been there once before, and it already felt like a second home to me. Once I walked through those doors, the pace of life slowed and I was transplanted to another universe. One where I feel more than comfortable. It reinforced my belief that I am living a calmer life. Calmer than the world out there. That I am staying balanced despite the trauma.

The woman who checked us in wore a flowing dress and strands of beads and had a silky, soothing voice that instantly relaxed me. She gave my friend and I our keys and, in our room, we unloaded our bags, then made our way to the healing arts spa to receive our massages. Afterward, we enjoyed a delicious vegetarian dinner where we met new and old friends.

The program we'd signed up for started on Friday night and led us through Sunday afternoon. Tucked away in an old converted monastery chapel, 230 women sat cross-legged on the floor, lightly clothed in the sweltering heat, inches away from other participants next to us, in front of us, and behind us. For hours, we sat in deep meditation, chanting mantras, singing, doing yoga, visualizing, tapping, and listening to soothing music. The leader of the session was a motivational leader who has been on Oprah and Dr. Oz and written five books. Throughout the weekend, she shared stories of her own struggles, to prove, she told us, that there is a "way through every block."

At one point, she stopped us and said, "I would like to open for Q and A." A dozen or more hands flew up. She called on them one by one, and they poured their hearts out to her, begging for her guidance as I observed and listened.

The first girl was about my age. I admired her dress and her shiny hair and strong body. She spoke softly but articulately. At first I thought she was going to tell an uplifting story, but I soon realized she was recounting her childhood rape by her brother and a life since plagued with humiliation and guilt.

The next girl stood up and described a troubled marriage where she felt she had no options: if she left she would lose her kids and money; if she stayed she would live with an abusive sociopath.

A third girl, a gentle girl, told about her lifelong struggle with a depression that was resistant to medication and she had frequent suicidal thoughts.

And then Olivia, sweet Olivia, a small blond sitting next to me whom I'd talked to over lunch. When she was 19 and living in Nepal, she was held up at gunpoint and raped, and when she later told someone about it, he was murdered. Fifteen years later she was still walking around in a fog of shame and grief.

Suddenly I felt the energy in the room change. I looked around to find our serene group of women becoming fearful, angry, and trauma-filled. One moment we were meditating together; the next, people were crying. There was a collective call for help, and it was loud.

But I remained calm. I watched myself stay clear and strong. As I had listened to each story, instead of thinking about my own problems, I focused on these women, one at a time. Their stories horrified me, but I didn't lose myself. In fact, I began to feel gratitude that my problems weren't that bad. I had money and health insurance, a happy childhood, a loving family. My heart went out to them.

Then the leader told a story of a girl who had the same name as me: Shanna. She said that four years ago, this Shanna was a participant at the same retreat and that she had an incurable form of cancer. Shanna was so happy to be there despite her poor prognosis and physical limitations. She recalled how everyone had formed a healing circle around Shanna and prayed for her and sang to her. Two weeks later, she died. She told us that if Shanna could find grace, so could we all.

I looked up, confused. Was she talking about me? I am, after all, Shanna, and I have an incurable form of cancer. Did someone tell her my story? Nope, Shanna died and I was here. Was she predicting what would happen to me? I didn't think so. What struck me most was that, again, I'd barely flinched when she told the story. Was I numb? Or had I reached a new level of inner strength and resilience? Yes, I confirmed, it was a feeling a freedom. I was experiencing an out of body phenomena.

I have had plenty of low points during my cancer journey — depression, anger, endless crying, and utter despair. But it has been quite some time since I felt sorry for myself. Years since I was so sad that I couldn't function. I have come a long, long way. In some ways, it feels like someone else's story now. I have moved in a different direction. I am living out a beautiful life of tranquility and grace. I am sure of it.

Sincerely,
Shanna

August 2017

Dear Universe,

Last night I told a friend that I am spiritual. "What do you believe?" she asked.

I said, "Well, I am Jewish and proud to be a Jew, but spiritually I have my own beliefs. I believe that I am part of something much bigger than myself and my tradition. I believe in love and faith, and that if I completely surrender, the stars will align and my life will unfold in divine time."

She looked at me like I was a little crazy.

Maybe that's what happens when you have progressions almost every year.

Every time I go into the cancer center for my PET scan results, I cross my left fingers and hold my breath. Sometimes I know it's coming because of symptoms I have been having or because I have been watching the tumor markers rise on the cancer center's online portal.

But when the words are spoken, it brings a visceral reaction every time. A feeling of utter and complete terror, and continued disbelief.

"You have grown multiple tumors up and down your spine and into your pelvis."

"You had a modest response to that treatment but the cancer is growing and it is time to move on to the next one."

"There is a new hormone medication that I think will address this."

"It's enough. I have used up the hormone treatments. This is a sign. It's time for chemo."

"Something is not working optimally. Let's get a bone biopsy."

"There is a very small suspicious spot in your lungs. We need to add a drug to your cocktail.

We have been at this for years. How is it still a complete shock when these words are spoken?

About a year ago, my spiritual rituals solidified. I decided that to live fully and peacefully with what I was going through, I needed to infuse spirituality into my life, and, after trying multiple avenues, I arrived at a practice.

It starts at the beginning of each new day. Truth be told, I have never been a morning person. For decades when my alarm went off, I would shudder, press snooze twice, and eventually roll out of bed feeling sick to my stomach and dreading the day. I wouldn't truly wake up for hours. I still press snooze, but now I play a song that I found on a Spotify station called "Amen." It is the sound of a woman saying thank you to you for another day. Her beautiful voice is filled with gratitude, respect, peace, and love. I fold over forward in prayer or I lie on my back with my hands up towards the sky as I think about how lucky I am to be alive.

It happens again in the afternoon. In the past, I never thought about taking a break from my busy day. I would go from school to activities to homework, from work to family responsibilities to social outings with friends. I still have very busy days, designing the interiors of homes, playing tennis, painting, and managing our hectic home life. But now, like clockwork, I take a break around 2pm. First I diffuse essential oils into the air. Then I lie on my side in a fetal position and play an Indian chant I also found on Spotify. The music is repetitive, deep and soulful. It takes me to another dimension. Sometimes I fall asleep for about 20 minutes. Then I wake up, have a cup of tea, and move on.

Every month or so I see my reiki master. I update her on my life and then lie on her table. She puts her hands on my chakras and channels grace and energy from the universe to me. I believe that she is truly doing that. I usually fall asleep on her table and when I wake up, she tells me what was clogged, what I needed from the universe and why. I always feel lighter when I leave her house.

Each summer I have what I call a spiritual cleansing. I seek out seminars and retreat centers to learn from. At these programs, I meet like-minded people who have all been through trauma – divorce, rape, losing a loved one, loneliness, depression, illness. I connect with them, and together we connect with you, dear universe. I try to absorb the healing messages that are dispersed in these sessions and keep them present in my life through intentions, affirmations, daily meditation practices, crystal jewelry, sculptures of Buddha, and light flowing clothing.

I admit, though, that sometimes the messages don't resonate. This year I am struggling with surrender versus intent as it relates to my health.

If I surrender to you completely, will you heal me? After all, only you know the course and timing of my disease. I have learned that my fate is much bigger than me. That there is only so much I can do to affect the outcome. I need to relax into that uncertainty and be grateful for each day and moment. And have faith.

But I have a strong intent to stay healthy and alive. Can this help my chances? Can I create my own reality? Isn't everything we are experiencing today a result of all the decisions we have made in the past? Maybe I am alive because I sent the right messages to my body. Because I got the best doctor. Because I removed a lot of stress from my lifestyle. At what point will it all come crashing down, like it has in the past?

Here is what am I afraid of: Missing out. Losing myself. Leaving my family. Feeling physical pain. Seeing others in pain.

Live in the moment. Let it be. Love. Accept. Blah, blah, blah. It's so easy to overthink these positive healing messages.

So, I ask the essential question. Who am I? I am more than a former VP at a big company, an interior designer, a mother, a wife, a daughter, a sister, a cancer patient wearing a bright yellow survivor shirt on scan day. I am a living and breathing soul, bringing happiness to myself and others, spreading light and love, helping the community around me to be a better place, a more creative place, a more authentic place.

And so, I settle back and I remind myself:

Don't force an outcome.

Embrace uncertainty.

When it feels right, it is.

Trust the unknown.

Be in alignment with the universe.

Sincerely,
Shanna

August 2018

Dear Universe,

It's been a while since we have spoken. I guess I am feeling like I need to check in. To make sure we are still aligned.

The treatments go on and on. I am mostly used to being on medication all the time.

I will admit that the side effects are getting harder to deal with. I try to tell myself that this is just physical and that I am still the same spirit. Just ignore the swollen red hands and feet, the pain in the hip, the fatigue and the reflux. These are little things in the grand scheme of you, right?

My meditation practice is going strong. I believe it is a form of prayer. I play the song "Amen" each morning. My older daughter knows every word and sings along with me. It's so cute. Then she will catch herself saying some strange phrase and ask me, "What is this weird song, Mommy?"

I try to squeeze in those 20-minute afternoon chanting meditations as well. Now my daughters and I meditate together before bed too. They love it and I can see their bodies relax into peace and serenity.

I visit my reiki master regularly for chakra rebalancing. I wear essential oils on my pressure points and diffuse oils to change my mindset and moods. And I just went to an ashram, my happy place, for a day in the Berkshires.

Yoga is part of my weekly routine when I am physically able to do it. I bow down in the rhythmic flow of sun salutations and feel an instant sense of serenity, like the old Sanskrit texts prescribed.

And this year I made two spiritual pilgrimages, one to Japan, where I immersed myself in Zen Buddhism and the spirit in nature, and then to Israel, where I felt embraced in the land of my own religion and history. India awaits, if I can find someone to go with me.

When I am in these spiritual spaces, my mind is alive and strong. I am living fully in the present. I am not thinking about my messed up past or my uncertain future. I am happy. I am peaceful. I am aware of my connection to you, Universe.

This was not always so. Now, as I move into the fifth year of my Stage Four illness, I want to talk to you about what has changed in my perspective.

For one thing, I recognize that "being spiritual" – consciously being aligned with you – is an invaluable tool for trauma. And I am certain that I have found the best set of spiritual practices that help me.

I believe every person should strive to do the same, and not blindly follow a framework that has been forced on them and may not suit them.

For example, maybe you are a Jewish person like me whose family has followed certain traditions for generations – like the ones that include holiday fasting; Shabbat prohibitions on using electricity, spending money and driving; Kosher eating that forbids shellfish and mixing milk and meat. Maybe you feel obliged to continue that path. But what if you don't agree with or understand the rules? What if you don't "feel" them the way you want to? Is it okay to create your own combination of beliefs and practices? Is it okay to look to other religions and pick and choose what works for you and only you?

I say yes. I encourage it. It has worked quite well for me. I don't believe in the restrictions of Jewish life, but I am happy that my kids go to Hebrew school and are learning about thousands of years of history and holidays that are still celebrated with as much vigor today. With my illness, the passage of time marked with Shabbat and all the annual holidays feel that much more meaningful and powerful now that I have a serious illness. My family and I celebrate each one that we can with excitement.

But ultimately, I would like them to explore a variety of belief systems and mix in other practices that resonate with them. I write this now so that one day they will understand this wisdom and know that I support their investigation of other traditions so that they can discover their own purpose and rituals. And that includes no rituals at all, if that is what they choose.

I want to tell them not to follow others blindly, even their family. I want them to find their own truths. Their own connections to you.

I grew up in an atheistic and rational household that valued facts over spirituality, science over religion, tangible proofs over a faith in G-d. It wasn't until I became ill that I began to reconsider this. It was my illness that urged me to seek out the beliefs and rituals that make me feel better. That help me and my family live more fully. That bring me closer to your energy, Universe, and the power I get from you that enriches my life.

I was taught that when you die, you are no more. You are buried under the ground. All that is left of you are pictures and memories that live on in others.

It was not until I was diagnosed with a terminal illness that I began to think about death and what will happen afterwards. And I realized I don't like the approach I was taught.

So, I decided to change it.

When I die, my spirit will rise into the clean, crisp air and hover over you, Universe, in a force so electric that it may change the weather or the colors in the sunset. Then it will disperse slowly and start to break apart. Each piece will be absorbed by someone I knew and loved. Different people will get different pieces. Some people will get the same pieces. Some people will get multiple pieces. These pieces will become part of their spirits. And change them forever.

And when they die, their spirits will be diffused into the atmosphere and into the people they loved.

Doesn't that sound beautiful?

It was not until I was diagnosed with a terminal illness that I began to think about hope and miracles. Medically, I know my disease is textbook: the cancer grows and is treated until there are no more treatments, and then it grows out of control and damages my organs until I die. There are statistical models that show the effectiveness of each treatment. There are statistical models that show my likelihood of making it two years, five years, 10 years. Yes, I appreciate the treatments and know they are keeping me alive. But I realized I didn't like the medical model.

So, I decided to change it.

After I have endured years and years of disease progression; of countless doctor appointments, injections, and IV infusions; of pills and scans and side effects; years and years of fatigue and pain and torture, there will be one more treatment. There will be no side effects. And it will cure me forever. Doesn't that sound beautiful?

Sincerely,
Shanna

June 2018

Dear Customer Service Representative,

You are the first person I've encountered inside the large bureaucracy of the 9/11 victim's agencies who has a brain.

And a heart.

Two years ago, I found out that if you have cancer, and were present at Ground Zero on 9/11, and returned to work at the World Financial Center "too early," you are eligible for victim compensation. A light bulb went on in my head. I immediately decided that my breast cancer had to have been caused by the terrorist attacks. If the studies pointed towards it, and there was no other reason behind my illness, then this was surely the culprit.

It made perfect sense. For years after the attacks, I held my breath when I walked into the office because the air was still thick and caught in my throat. My eyes burned. I was nervous and called the health department, where someone told me that tests had been performed and the air was clean; it was safe to work there, they assured me. Employee communications went out in my company with similar information. But I knew something was wrong.

For two years, I have been filling out forms, signing papers, faxing and mailing packages into a big dark hole called the September 11th Victim Compensation Fund. I have their phone number on my speed dial. I've spoken to dozens of customer service reps who never provided their names, never had any information, and certainly never helped me. "Go to the website," they all said curtly. I followed whatever directions I could find online and hoped I would hear back.

I didn't think there was anyone there who cared. I didn't think there was anyone there who could guide me. I didn't think anyone was going to recognize me as injured from the terrorist attacks, or that I could receive the validation or compensation I deserved.

I don't know why I kept pushing for it. Yes, it gave me purpose, but for the bullshit I was dealing with, I should have given up months before. But I didn't.

Despite placing weekly calls to try and move the process along, I heard nothing for almost a year. Until one day I received a letter from the World Trade Center Health Program directing me to go to Long Island for a checkup.

So, I called (again).

"Hello," you said. "How may I help you?"

It was the first time I heard a friendly voice.

"What's this all about?" I asked.

You paused briefly as you looked over my files. "Yes," you said, "this is the next step. It's easy: just go and give them some blood and some urine, and hopefully we can get you certified. You will probably have to talk to another doctor who can link your condition to the terrorist attacks. But it's moving forward."

"You mean I can actually get certified?" I asked.

"Yes, keep at it," you said.

"Thanks. It is so much easier when there is a human being to talk to," I told you.

And with that I launched into my entire story, from the panic of the 9/11 attacks, to the agonies of being sick with cancer. I pleaded for your help. And you listened, clicking away on your computer.

The next week my dad drove me to Long Island. I had driven through this town countless times during my childhood. It was a dingy neighborhood that connected my town to another nearby affluent town with a huge shopping mall. I was always fascinated passing the dirty streets lined with rambling buildings and littered with homeless people, and then crossing an invisible border where everything suddenly transformed into manicured homes and stores. We had never stopped in the town in between. But this time we had to go straight to the center of it.

I had brought my dad for protection because I wasn't sure what to expect. We parked outside the building and took the elevator to the 11th floor, the Industrial Health Department. A woman checked us in. We sat in the overly-bright waiting room with chairs around the perimeter and a blaring television. There were a few others waiting, too.

When my name was called, I went back to see a nurse who barely spoke English. I knew she wanted to take blood, and I explained that I am a hard stick because my veins are shot from chemo. Might they have special valves and heat packs? She looked at me like I was crazy and called another nurse. It took over an hour for them to draw my blood. I was nauseous – but again felt that sense of determination. After I peed in a cup, they said they wanted some chest X-rays.

"Why?" I asked.

"It's part of the process," they barked.

I speed-dialed the Victim Compensation Fund on my cell phone, and you picked up. "Hello," you said. I recognized your voice.

"It's me," I said, as if you would know who I was out of the hundreds of thousands of applicants. "They want me to have an unnecessary X-ray."

You knew exactly who I was. "Decline it. Don't worry. It doesn't matter."

The next week I got a letter with instructions to see a doctor in New Jersey. I called you, and you explained that this was another necessary step.

This time my husband drove me. To an equally seedy neighborhood in New Jersey.

I filled out paperwork and waited to be seen.

A doctor with a strong Russian accent poked and prodded me and asked me about any symptoms I might have experienced since my exposure to the fumes of 9/11.

"Let me walk you through my story," I stated. She made a few notes and then dismissed us.

A week later I called, and you picked up again. Amazing.

You explained that you were my case specialist. That all the information was in and that the final step was for you to summarize the findings and submit them to the government. "I really want you to get certified," you said. "The evidence is clear."

It didn't matter that we were on a recorded line. I felt like I was talking to a friend.

"The only catch is timing," you continued. "There are thousands of people like you waiting to get certified, many without any health coverage, and there are only seven of us here. You have my commitment to expedite this, but I don't know how long it will take on the government side. I feel for you."

"Just do your best," I told him. I knew I was in good hands.

A month later I got a voicemail from you. I heard the excitement in your voice. You urged me to call you back as soon as possible.

I had you paged. "What's going on?" I asked.

"You are certified," you said. "We just found out. We got the fax from the government minutes ago. You're in!"

I didn't know exactly what this meant even though I had been pushing for it for years.

"The government has recognized that the 9/11 terrorist attacks caused your cancer. It means that you never will have to worry about health care costs like co-pays again. And although it is another lengthy process, you are eligible for compensation."

"How difficult is that to get?" I asked.

"Very," you said. "Applicants have to be persistent. Like you. And because there are so few of us to advocate for you and only a handful of reviewers, it can take years. To give you an idea, there are 10,000 applicants in process. You deserve this. You need this."

"Thanks," I said.

Yes. I deserve this. I expect to get compensated for all the damages done to me. But mostly I feel a sense of closure. Like my story is unfolding. The events of my life are starting to make sense.

Thanks for reminding me that it is the human heart that perseveres.

Sincerely,
Shanna

GET OUT OF YOUR STRESSFUL JOB

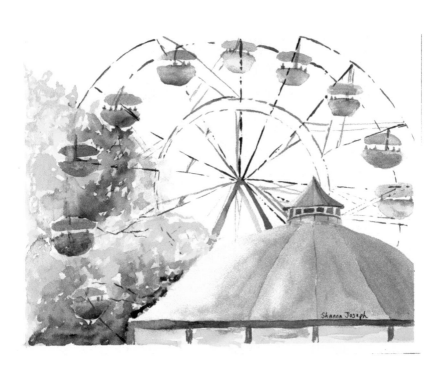

February 2015

Dear Company,

Today, after more than 14 years, I left my job working for you. I was your employee in many capacities, but most recently as VP and Head of North American Marketing. Fourteen years of building credentials, expertise, an extensive network, "executive presence", and a solid reputation. Moving up higher and higher. And just like that, a chapter has ended. A major turn around the corner has happened, my hair whipping with the wind. Hard to believe.

Amazing how it takes a serious illness to finally give myself permission to do exactly what I want. Not because it will earn me an A, get me into an Ivy League college, land me a good job, or find me a nice Jewish boy to marry. Not because my doctor told me to. But simply because I want to experience life and feel alive.

After the Stage Four diagnosis, I told my boss I couldn't go on. For weeks, I felt like I had been torn in half. My career was part of me, it ran through my blood. But it had never been clearer that I had to leave to focus on my health. My boss had seen what I had been through and agreed that it was the right decision. "You have to take care of yourself first," he said, and for the first time, I saw a glimmer of humanity in a man I'd always considered a serious workaholic.

The arrangement was that I would stay through February. The announcement would be made at the end of December. So, for the rest of the Fall I pretended like nothing was wrong. It was business as usual. Although my head was not even close to there. Then after the announcement was made in December I read the look of shock on my colleagues' faces. Were they really surprised? I clearly had health issues. I was in and out of the office. I looked like hell. But they were. I thought I could hear people whispering around me in the hallways: "Did her cancer return? Is it too much for her to handle? Does she not care anymore? Was she fired?" How refreshing that I couldn't care less what people thought. I was out of there.

I cleaned out my office, had some final lunches, listened in on meetings, and helped here and there. I left with a handful of personal items including an office placard with my name on it, which I proudly placed on my desk in our kitchen.

It seems like yesterday that I dropped my resume in your slot for on-campus recruiting in the fall of 1999. This was the beginning of another one of life's rides. I wanted a good job badly. I had a degree in Communications and Marketing and had my sights set on working at a big brand. When you called me in for a day of interviews a week later, I was nervous because technically I wasn't in business school, and I wasn't sure I was qualified. But the woman across the table was smiling and pleasant, and we hit it off immediately. My passion came through in our early discussions. The next thing I knew, you called to invite me to the headquarters to meet some of the senior leaders. You put me up in a hotel and took me out for fancy meals. I got my offer in the mail a couple of weeks later, and it was signed before Thanksgiving. A sign-on bonus was transferred to my bank account, and two free air tickets to Europe were sent to my house as a congratulatory gift. My parents were proud. I was excited. Our relationship was off to a good start.

My first job was as an Analyst on a newly launched credit card. I had no idea what anyone was talking about. Many people had MBAs and multiple years of experience. I clung to my comrades, who had also been recruited from undergraduate programs, and, thankfully my boss took me under her wing and nurtured me.

Every two years I would move from one job to another within your organization. That made the time fly, because there were always new skills to learn and new people to meet. I would master the role I was in, launch some big product or program, do some networking, and then get either promoted or relocated to another division.

I had plenty of tough times. Colleagues whom I couldn't stand. Bosses who could be confusing. Political battles and people who stabbed me in the back. Hundreds of PowerPoint presentations and Excel spreadsheets. Too many deadlines. So many bumps but always moving right on up.

I never once thought about leaving you. Every morning I got a large coffee and breakfast in the cafeteria to start my day. Before I knew it, I had worked on more partnerships, new products, loyalty programs, analytical programs, strategies, branding, communications, and P&Ls than I could count. I was building skills that helped me to become an expert, a leader in the company, a marketing guru.

As the years passed, I noticed the employees getting younger. The senior leaders left and new ones were appointed. Thousands of people were laid off, and you reorganized, reorganized again, and then reorganized once more. My title was upgraded, and in 2012 I got my first office. I had 15 people reporting to me. I dressed in suits and fancy heels and spoke with confidence to some of the top executives at the company. I had arrived.

I will never forget today. My last day. The day my boss walked me out of your building. He walked me to the turnstiles and stopped so that I could give him my badge and he could give me a hug. And as I walked through those turnstiles, I felt something lift from my shoulders. I felt lighter as I headed to the subway, so much so that I started running, and my heart started racing, and I realized that I could slow down because I wasn't going anywhere but home. I liked my job, but mostly I liked the way it made me feel accomplished and important. How people looked at me and complimented my outfits, watched me as I absorbed what we were talking about in a meeting and waited for my input on a decision. It made me feel successful when people asked me what I did for a living and I said I ran the marketing department.

But what was I really doing anyway? Not much, I'm afraid. From the outside of your company now, I am convinced we were just talking to ourselves in all those meetings, and often in circles. We were "increasing revenue," "growing the business," "strengthening the brand," but looking back, it all feels so intangible. I never really saw any of those things or even cared. It was the ego driving those discussions: money and power, not a greater purpose or intention to help anyone but ourselves. Now I see that that was what was missing for me. Not to mention all the weeks and days and hours it sucked away from my personal life and my family. Two weeks after my departure, you threw a going-away party for me with lots of food and drinks and laughter. My now-ex-coworkers toasted me – "a friend to everyone." But it already felt different. Interesting that it's been months and not one of those people has called to see how their friend is doing.

Fortunately, because of my disability checks, I think I will be able to choose how to spend my time, and one of the first things I learned was that life goes on.

I will become more involved in the kids' lives than ever before. I will know exactly what activities are happening each day, who is being mean to whom on the playground, and who needs new underwear and sneakers before the old ones get too small. The girls and I will go ice skating weekly in the winter, and to the pool in the summer. I will cook delicious meals for my husband and me. Our refrigerator will be filled with fresh fruits and vegetables instead of frozen food and take-out.

I will see my parents often, for lunch or for walks. We will talk about how they are doing, the new friends they have made since they moved, what is new with the kids. When I am tired, my mom will make me lunch and rub my feet. When I am anxious, she will tell me I will be fine, and I will believe her. My dad will drive me to treatments when I need help and fix things in the house for me.

I will get certified in interior design, because I have always wanted to decorate other people's homes – and my own. I will take watercolor classes and build my own portfolio. I will frame my paintings around the house. They will reflect the beautiful world around me.

When it rains, or is cold outside, I will sleep late, then snuggle under the covers and watch TV. When it clears up, I will have tea in my garden and then walk around the corner to stare at the water. Heavenly! I will work out, meditate, feel and look good. For the first time in my life, I will dye my hair blond and straighten it too, just as I always dreamed of it being.

And I will write my book. I always wanted to write a book but never had the time. Or the patience. And I thought I didn't have content that was interesting enough. Well here it is: my life, real time. More content than I know what to do with.

How drastically different everything is today from what it was a couple of years ago. Some days I don't recognize myself in the mirror. My corporate wardrobe has been given away to charities or hidden in the attic. Those bags under my eyes are pretty much erased. I can wear whatever I want. I can do what I want. I can say what I want. I can take deeper breaths.

Yes, the disease is there. It will require lots of time and management, with constant visits to the doctor's office, daily medications, blood draws, infusions and injections every three weeks, PET scans every four months, nagging side effects like nausea, diarrhea, insomnia, and low blood counts. But I will hide most of that from the rest of the world, at least for now. I prefer it that way. That is the easy stuff. I think about it like a part time job.

Interestingly, it will be my disease that will give me the power to be happy and at peace. This is also not visible to the outside world. I will have the awareness to know that every second of every day is precious. There is no time to waste. I will jump on every opportunity that sounds interesting to me. Frankly, I do whatever I want, whenever I want. The highs will be higher than ever.

What if everyone chose to design their own lives? People talk about "when they retire" or "when the kids are older," but what if they knew they didn't have that luxury?

Because maybe they don't. Because life is uncertain for everyone, and there is no time to waste. The time is now. It is always now.

Sincerely,
Shanna

December 2017

Dear Diary,

My British boss always called the schedule, or the calendar, a "diary." I thought it was so cute. As if it were a thoughtful book of events, instead of a jumbled mess of stressful responsibilities.

There were about 21 months, between my Stage Two and Stage Four diagnoses, when we thought I was cured. When the likely outcome was that I would recover physically and emotionally from all the treatments I had been through and put it all behind me. When we thought that the cancer would shrink into the past, smaller and smaller until it disappeared. We believed I would be able to return to how things had been with you, dear diary, and get on with my life.

The plan was that I would go to the doctor frequently for a couple years, then less and less, until I would "graduate" from the cancer center. I would "revive" my old life, and my kids would grow up without ever knowing that I had once been sick.

Unfortunately, that didn't happen. But for 21 months, all of us (including my doctors, my boss and my colleagues, my parents and siblings, my husband) thought it would.

During that time, I tried to resume my old routines. I went back to work after taking a nine-month sick leave. And within a couple of weeks, you were filled to the brim again, just like you had been before my first diagnosis.

Every morning, I woke up to the sound of the alarm and pressed snooze. While waiting for it to sound again, I pictured my day and envisioned myself in various outfits. I got up with care so as not to wake the girls. I put on uncomfortable pants or a skirt and a tailored shirt or sweater; I always added a chunky necklace or an interesting pair of shoes to add some personality, a little bit of foundation and eye makeup, and I was ready to go. Breakfast would have to wait. My babysitter walked in as I walked out, and I told her the kids were still sleeping.

I remember my first day back: there I was again, as if I had never left. My car parked at the station, me on the Metro-North platform. The same guy standing next to me while we waited for the train to arrive. Everyone, including me, checking their phones through their dark sunglasses. Once we boarded, I made myself comfortable in a front-facing window seat and connected my headphones to my Spotify morning playlist. I turned on my Blackberry and checked you once or twice to try and mentally prepare for the day. When we got to Grand Central, I was almost asleep, abruptly awakened by the blare of the conductor announcing our arrival.

I stepped off the train into the masses seemingly walking into one another. I knew the most efficient way to the Four train. Sunglasses still on my face, headphones still on my ears, I descended downwards on the escalators and then down again into the depths of the underground city.

It usually took two trains to come and go before there was enough room for me to get on, and the same was true on that day. I pressed myself against the pole and closed my eyes against the creepy guy on one side of me and the screaming baby in the arms of an exasperated woman on the other. Through my headphones, I could hear the alerts of the subway stops as we made our way downtown. I changed my playlist to something more fast-paced to match my heart rate.

When we got downtown, it was almost 8:45am. People began pushing one another forcefully to get out of the train and then the station and make a beeline for their desks before the 9 o' clock hour. I felt myself being lifted by the crowds; I always wondered if

I could simply let them carry me along. According to you, I had to get in by 9am, too.

Once outside, I wiped the beads of sweat off my forehead and looked around at the tall buildings, trying to get my bearings, even though I had done this a thousand times. Oh, right: across Ground Zero in a single-file line, one New Yorker after another, all with blank and somewhat annoyed expressions on their faces. Then across the street, up the escalator, fingerprint on the turnstile, and another wait at the elevator bank. Pushing myself into the elevator, I knew I was late, and my heart started racing. I ran to my office, threw off my coat, grabbed some papers off my desk, and rushed to where I thought the meeting was but wasn't exactly sure.

My colleagues were waiting in the conference room for the stragglers. Someone dialed in, and the meeting began. Once I sat down, I could rest for a couple of minutes. I nodded profusely as if I were listening to what was being said. I worried that I would be asked a question, because frankly I had no idea what we were talking about. I discreetly checked you on my Blackberry under the table and then silently gasped as I realized that I was back-to-back until 1:30pm. Food, and any type of thoughtful planning, was going to have to wait.

Between the nine and ten o'clock meetings, my boss found me and called me into his office. There was a group of people gathered around his small conference table debating about an "issue" that had come up and had to be resolved immediately. I wasn't exactly up to speed and tried to pay attention, but my brain was like mush. All I could tell was that someone had dropped the ball, and everyone was attacking him. One colleague was showing off her grasp of the situation and coming up with "innovative" ideas. Another colleague was the fact checker and had a pile of papers that she was referencing, trying to prove her knowledge. I knew

I was missing some other meeting and wondered how important that one was and if they would even notice that I wasn't there.

When I finally came in, a woman on my team was showcasing a recent marketing launch. I felt a glimmer of pride as I scanned the images on the screen and thought back to when this campaign had been just an idea. Now it was in the marketplace. Customers were interacting with the program and showing interest. Our business partners were thrilled. We were getting the credit we deserved.

The day passed in a blink. I remember at some point running to the cafeteria to grab pre-made sushi from the refrigerator, and at another point running down to Starbucks for some caffeine. I tried to organize the papers on my desk into what had to get done today and what could wait until tomorrow, Friday, next week, next month. The numbers of red unread emails in my inbox were increasing.

I thought briefly about when and how I was going to exercise this week and couldn't come up with any options. Maybe over the weekend.

My husband texted me a one-word "hi" in the middle of the day. I didn't have time to respond.

I thought about checking in with the babysitter to see how the kids' days were and if my elder daughter still had a sniffle. Which activity were they at now? I checked you to find out. At the same moment, I saw an email come in from an old friend with dates for getting together; we have been trying for months to nail something down. Also at the same moment I realized I was late for my next meeting.

During the 4pm meeting, I was called back into my boss's office. There was another "issue" that needed our attention. There we sat at his conference table coming up with a plan. This one entailed flying out to San Francisco in the next week to meet with the partner and address a misconception. I pulled you up and tried to see what could be moved around both personally and professionally. There were too many doctors' appointments. I was going to have to bow out. I was disappointed. A woman sitting next to me whispered in my ear that she couldn't take it anymore. She was "done." I agreed with sympathy.

Suddenly you reminded me that it was past 5pm and I needed to go. The end of the meeting was nowhere in sight, so I looked around awkwardly, made a few final remarks, and said that I had to leave to relieve the babysitter. I ran out of the office and into the night. I felt guilty, unaccomplished, and alone. I felt so far away from home.

The commute home was always painful. I was exhausted and barely aware of my surroundings. I was too distracted to read or catch up on the news. I stared blindly out the train window into the darkness.

When I got home, the kids jumped all over me. Although happy to see them, I felt oddly violated. I needed to get out of my clothes and into my pajamas immediately, I thought. The babysitter was already out the door. "Mommy come color with me," "Mommy I want to watch more TV." Their voices got louder and louder on top of each other. My husband was nowhere to be found.

Somehow in the next hour, I was made comfortable, my husband came home, and the kids were pacified and put to bed. It was a complete blur. I moved like I was in a dream, on autopilot. The house was a mess. My husband would binge-watch TV downstairs late into the night to relax, while I passed out in minutes. The next day, it all started again.

And what did I have to show for it? The days turned into weeks, the weeks turned into months, the months turned into years. I was supposed to be grateful.

Then came the Stage Four diagnosis, and everything changed. Within months I left my job. I still used you to manage my life, dear diary, but now you're on my iPhone (my Blackberry was turned in with my security badge). And now the only things that get added to you are by me, not my assistant. I don't have an assistant.

At first, there were lots of medical appointment to manage. And lots of open spots for naps. Although I hated seeing what used to be slots for meetings now filled with doctors' names, I realized that, unlike ever before, I was taking care of myself as a priority.

Once the cancer was under control, my days – and your slots – started to change. I began to plan my life. This time forever, not a sick leave.

Now I wake up about an hour later than before, sometimes to the sound of the alarm, but more often to the sound of one of my daughters going to the bathroom or coming into my bedroom. We listen to music in the morning, and we scratch each other's backs. We hug a lot.

After we get dressed, in comfortable clothes for us all, we go downstairs. I make my girls' breakfast and pack them snacks and lunch. I do one of my daughter's hair. I write notes to their teachers, gather up their library books, and zip their backpacks. The house is quiet and warm. The sun of the new day is coming in through our light-filled family room. The girls' laughter and little voices fill the air. I love every second of it all.

During the drive to school, I usually check you and tell the girls what they can expect later in the day: who has what activities and play dates and sports and where. The babysitter helps with the driving and the dinner prep. But you and I, dear diary, are the ones who do the planning. The ones who organize how my girls' will spend their time, who arrange their growing lives. We do with deliberation and care. Proactive, not reactive.

After I drop them off, I go home for a well-deserved meeting with me, myself, and I. We usually sit in front of the Today show with some hot tea and breakfast. We put you aside while we slowly become more alert. More and more interested in what the hours will bring. And when we are ready, we go out and start our day.

Some are more focused on physical activities, like walks in the woods, or personal training sessions at the gym, or tennis matches. Other days I run from store to store checking off errands and stocking the fridge with healthy fruits and veggies. At least a couple of days a week, I am involved in the interior design work that I have taken on – whether through real projects or class work. And once a week, I take out my watercolors and paint with a group of likeminded artists, all of us focused on how the colors and shapes come alive.

I check you multiple times a day. And if I don't like the way we are set up, I press "edit delete" or "edit reschedule." If I am tired, I schedule a nap and head home. A few times a week I fit in a few hours to prepare healthy meals for me and my family.

When the girls come home, we read, snuggle on the couch, watch TV, and do art projects. They tell me about their days and their friends, and sometimes they tell me about what they are learning.

At night, occasionally I will disappear and have dinner with a friend. On the weekends, my husband and I make dates with other couples or attend parties. We keep the house clean and tidy and the refrigerator stocked. The bills are paid before they turn into a scary stack.

My wardrobe, too, has changed. From structured to casual. The materials softer and more comfortable. The jewelry more trendy than fancy. My high heels now sit in the back of my closet, and I have a whole new suite of sandals and cool boots. The remaining suits and dresses have become my annual attire for Rosh Hashanah services.

When I think about it, my days and weeks and months are just as jam-packed.

But my concerns are utterly different.

I wonder how the kids are going to have time for ice skating when we are already doing so many sports. I wonder how we can go on three international trips this year, instead of two. I wonder if going out to four social events a week is too many, and what will I wear? I wonder if I can fit a design internship into my weeks when I am already committed to Tuesday painting groups. How will I choose between writing a book and starting a creative business of my own?

I know in my heart that if I hadn't received that devastating Stage Four diagnosis, I would still be commuting to the city and surviving blurry and nerve-wracking days – some, yes, gratifying, but most filled with repetition in that dry and stale office. My resume would grow from two pages, to three, and then four, with impressive new titles and accomplishments. The days would turn to weeks, and the weeks to months, and the months to years, and the years to decades. I know that before I knew it, the girls would be grown.

There would be trips that I didn't have time to take, friends who were lost because there wasn't enough time to stay in touch, a gnawing dissatisfaction that I had never explored my innermost creativity and expression, and, most devastating of all, an endless guilt that I didn't know my girls as well as I wanted to.

You would have been filled, dear diary. But with nothing that mattered.

Now, each year you are filled with a life worth living. We are packing it in. And you are the chronicle of it all. This is what I call a "diary."

Sincerely,
Shanna

May 2018

Dear Boss,

I woke up with a little more kick in my step. After I picked out the kids' clothing, instead of throwing on my usual sweatpants for school drop-off, I picked out clothing for me, too. Instead of my usual glasses and makeup-free face, I went into the bathroom and put on contacts, tinted moisturizer, lip gloss, and some mascara, and then I added a necklace. When I packed up the girls' backpacks, I packed up mine, too, with a new notebook, box of pencils, drawing paper, and my scale and tape measure. I was not going to design school. I was going to work!

My husband and I came up with the idea together. My semester was light – I must take just a few more classes to complete my certificate program, and none were offered this spring. So, I had the time.

But the thought of "going back to work" brought on a rush of emotions. I worried about putting myself back into a situation where I would feel stressed and out of control. I reminded myself that the hours would be limited to when my kids were in school, and I hoped that I had changed enough to respect my self-care needs. Let's do this, I thought.

I searched online and identified local design companies. Then I started networking until I whittled them down to a few prospects. I updated my resume and put together a portfolio, and there I was, interviewing, talking about myself as a designer. I had good references – from my old company and the director at my school. Now I have a three-day-a-week gig.

Who would have thought that a girl with metastatic breast cancer would reinvent her career?

I was in ninth grade when I started to think about what to do with my life. I knew it had to be creative, but I wondered what vocation would integrate that with my analytical, organized, Type A character. I eventually decided it was marketing (the "creative" form of business), and my 15-year run at it was indeed fulfilling. Plus, it made me a decent amount of money. But I never entirely grasped the corporate dynamic; it felt intangible, uncomfortable, out of reach.

It wasn't until I was diagnosed with breast cancer that I considered interior design as my true calling. Suddenly it was clear as could be. It might have had something to do with timing: we'd just bought a new house. A blank slate of rooms. And a distraction from the rigorous treatments my health crisis required.

I found my mind drifting from chemotherapy to kitchens, from doctor appointments to fabrics. In six short months, every corner of my house was decorated, and I loved the results. It was my first time doing any of this – measuring, creating floor plans, shopping, picking fabrics, hanging art in just the right places. Now everything feels cozy and peaceful. It is home.

The living room has a world theme. It's where all our artifacts from traveling live, alongside gifts from friends who have traveled. The few pieces I have purchased from stores, including a fantastic piece of artwork over the mantel, are handmade in other countries like Bali, India, and the Philippines. The room is usually empty. Except for me. Sometimes I bring a blanket in there, turn on the salt lamp, and snuggle up on the studded couch. I was thinking of myself when I designed this room. It is like a museum, but one that I can live in and enjoy each day.

The bedroom is an oasis of serenity. I picked colors that relax me, which turned out to be a lack of color – different shades of white and taupe. I picked out every detail, down to the sheets on the bed and the mirror on the makeup vanity. When I go up there at the end of the day, I sink into tranquility. I love that years later I am still obsessed with the wallpaper and furniture I chose.

These are just two rooms in an entire house that I designed. For our family.

I dreamed of designing beautiful environments for others that would add comfort and joy to their lives. I found myself staring at other people's rooms, overlaying the future potential of these spaces onto their current state. That's when I enrolled in design school.

I knew my corporate life was over, and, given how driven I have always been, it was hard to do nothing. I welcomed my new endeavor. The school projects were challenging and time-consuming, but gratifying, and before I knew it, I was speaking the lingo of the trade, tossing off words like "elevations" and "scale," and learning the names of the popular brands like Stark and Kravet. I was also building my technical skills in drafting, pattern and color scheme. The days turned into weeks, the weeks into semesters, the semesters into years. Soon I will receive my certificate of completion. And even before that I have an actual job.

However.

I never told you about the breast cancer.

I also never told my teachers at design school or any of my peers.

There were days when I pushed myself to make the drive to school, some new medication causing crushing fatigue. There were weeks when I was so behind on projects that I considered telling the head of the design program that I had a "condition." But every time, I pushed through. I caught up, I studied, I read the material, I went on the field trips, I took the exams, I did the assignments, I put together huge client boards, and I presented my final projects.

One day, the head of the program, who also taught one of my classes, told us about a student who had a chronic illness (I think it was rheumatoid arthritis) and what a shame it was. This student struggled through her classwork, with his support, of course, but always fell short. Didn't finish a project, didn't finish a semester. She is still enrolled, and he prays that one day she will finish. She is so talented, he said. What a waste. What a poor, poor girl.

That is exactly why I never told anyone there about my illness. I knew it would change the way I was viewed – and the way I would view myself. I would always wonder if I were succeeding on my own merit or because I was special. I would always be slightly embarrassed.

My first day of work with you was terrific. We hit it off immediately, and I followed you around with a notebook on a job site as you dictated to me what was going on and what needed to get done. I dove in head first, providing my ideas but also trying to learn from you. What a coincidence that you also used to work in marketing, and that you were an artist before you went to school to become an interior designer.

The first week flew by. I met all the subcontractors. I met one of your clients. I felt like I was absorbing the content and already accomplishing.

Given how busy you are, I am not sure you noticed that the second, third, and fourth weeks were not as seamless. At least for me.

The second week was my PET scan, so I was preoccupied. I said goodbye to you one afternoon knowing that the next morning I would be waking up and driving to the cancer center to get my IV and drink my isotope drink. After 20 minutes in the machine, I would be free to go, but I would feel slightly nauseated, exhausted from the anti-anxiety pills, and nervous as could be.

We found out that it was a good scan and I could stay on my drug regimen. Hooray! But I still had to spend hours in waiting rooms and doctors' offices that week. Probably not what you envisioned me doing on my "day off."

The third week I discovered that the girls and I had lice. Our heads were itching like crazy – I kept telling myself it was the dry weather. But no. There were dozens of animals living on our scalps. I spent a week doing laundry, taking the kids for combings, communicating with the school and their friends. I was so upset that I left early one day. Just an hour early. I told you about the lice. It felt okay because it was a "mom" issue that I thought you could relate to. "Oh no!" you said in disbelief.

I was so exhausted that third week that I knew I was going to get sick. My outfits were not as cute as they had been the first week. I could barely get myself together. You were more comfortable having me around by then, I could tell. You threw more and more work my way. "Of course," I said. "Not a problem."

My kids had their talent show that week, and we went to practice every night. The younger had a cold and a cough, and the older was complaining of aches and pains, but we powered through. I picked out decorative pillows for one of your clients and she loved them.

The fourth week I fell apart. I had three doctors' appointments on my off days. I can do this, I thought. I drove to the city, saw the dermatologist about the rash on my face (blood capillaries growing as a side effect of my medications that were lasered off), saw my gynecologist to tell her that I got my period for the first time in five years (the look on her face was priceless, and I am still confused about what it means to have your period, go through menopause, be in menopause for five years, and then *not* be in menopause. I don't think she knows either!). I also saw the allergist to discuss the swollen itchy skin reactions I have been having since the summer. Probably from the chemo lowering your immunity, he said. We started patch testing; my back was covered in 300 stickers. No showering for a week, he said.

Then I found out my older daughter had fifth disease. Sounds more serious than it is. That's why she was aching and her face was bright red. We still went to her orchestra concert. And to the girls' talent show.

Afterwards I completely lost my voice. And I mean completely.

I showed up on Thursday to work like that. I have no idea why. I am not getting paid. I think I wanted to tell you in person that I wasn't well and couldn't work my hours, to "show" you instead of sending a text. That's my Type A ambitious self. You told me to do a couple of errands and then go get some rest. I whispered thanks and went home to bed.

I cancelled lunch with a friend. I cancelled my appointment with my trainer at the gym. Then I spent a couple of days on the couch, meditation music on and essential oils diffusing through the air. I sipped dozens of glasses of hot tea with honey and lemon. Thank G-d for my babysitter; she handled the kids and did the week's remaining errands.

But I still had to get up and go to the doctor on Friday. My husband and I waited for over an hour in the waiting room. Everyone was wearing a mask to prevent getting the flu. Once I was called to a room, the nurse poked me three times to find my vein, drew the usual four tubes of blood, and then hung the two bags of medications that would flow intravenously through my body for the next hour (Herceptin treatment). I watched the news while my husband checked sports and the market. By the time we left, I was so tired I felt like I was dreaming. He helped me get ready for bed and tucked me in. I slept for 12 hours straight.

It took months for me to feel better. To get more energy. I got many massages to ease my sore muscles. My voice came back, but it took so long that people noticed. The kids felt better, too. It was the usual hurricane. It passed, but it will come again.

I will try to shield you from the chaos of my life. I think it's best for us both. I just don't think you would be able to understand. I need to navigate this one by myself. It is my responsibility, not yours, to keep the stress out this experience.

And so, we continue our journey together, you, my new boss, and I, a 39-year-old mom with Stage Four breast cancer. I am excited. I will learn from you, and you will learn from me. I look forward to the amazing creations we will make together.

Thanks to you, I can see the future.

Sincerely,
Shanna

OPEN YOUR MIND

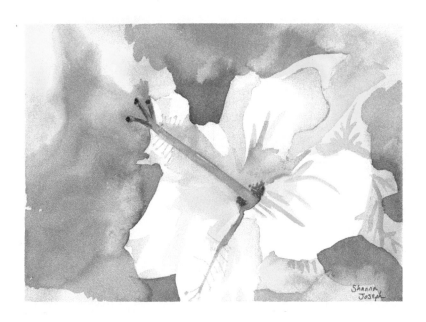

May 2015

Dear Stress and Fear,

Was it genetic? The effects of September 11th? Bad luck? The fertility treatments? There is no way to know why I got sick, but I believe that the toxic pair of you, Stress and Fear, had an important role.

Others may have been able to handle the mountains of stress I was under, but not me, and not my body.

Others may have been able to manage the pervasive fear of disease I carried, but not me, and not my body.

In retrospect, I can see how I got so caught up in stress, stress, and more stress. After all, I had set my sights high. I wanted to build a life in the New York area, and there is nothing easy about that. Nothing easy about fending for yourself in the big city, earning enough money to pay the rent, developing a career, making friends, trying to find a husband, building confidence, and, frankly, growing up.

I realize now that I had issues with you, Stress, at a very young age. Because I am not a naturally extroverted person, being a good student became the way to differentiate myself. This escalated quickly into a desire to be at the top of my class in a competitive large public school. A desire to get a high-paying corporate job. A desire for a house in the suburbs where I could raise a family. It never stopped.

I remember being at a swim meet in ninth grade, super anxious because I was going to get home late and I wasn't sure if I had prepared enough for my math test the next day. While the other girls swam, I hid in the locker room and studied. My mom found me there, and I can still see the look of concern on her face.

"Shanna, don't worry," she said quietly. "It's just a test. Now go out there and swim."

I also remember talking on the phone with my friends for hours, analyzing every detail of my life – every social situation, homework assignment, upcoming test, conflict with family members or other friends. Always so stressed. For decades. I think it would surprise most people that I worried so much, because I have a very calm demeanor. But it's the truth. You were always there.

As were you, Fear. In retrospect, I think I feared getting cancer from the time I was a small child. I don't know why, but I always thought that I was going to die young, and that it would be a tragic and awful death. I was also afraid that my mom was going to die or that my friends were going to die.

I remember watching the movie "Beaches," where the star's young mother dies of a heart disease. I cried my eyes out thinking this would happen to me. Then I watched the movie again and again and again.

I also remember a third-grade writing project where I wrote a story about a girl whose best friend dies of cancer. I wrote about the chemotherapy, the surgery, and the spread of the disease throughout her body. How I knew about such things at that age is beyond me.

For years, I was propelled to doctors' appointments thinking I had cancer, and they couldn't find anything wrong with me.

Stress and Fear, you were my constant companions. Until my diagnosis. Then our relationship changed. What I had worried about so urgently, so determinedly, no longer seemed as important.

Yes, we still need to feed our family, clean the dishes, and keep the lawn looking good. Yes, we still need to pay for our mortgage, not to mention my cancer meds. Topnotch health insurance is critical. My husband needs to keep his job or find another one.

We need to get along nicely with our extended family and the neighbors, and to do our best as we raise our daughters.

But these daily challenges aren't so heavy anymore. The anxiety has lifted. And I am no longer afraid of a cancer diagnosis because it has already happened. Once you have been told that your life will likely be cut short, the only thing that matters is to live.

So bye-bye, Stress and Fear. I can't help but blame you – at least a little – for my illness, and I'm happy to see you go. Everyone else might be plagued by worry. But not me.

Sincerely,
Shanna

August 2015

Dear Summer,

It's summer again. Another full circle. The air smells sweet, and I can feel the warmth of the sun on my skin. It is easier to breathe and for my muscles to relax.

Summer has always been my favorite season. Maybe because I hate the cold, or because people move a bit more slowly and are a little nicer. Maybe because it is when I was born, so it seems like a beginning.

It is an unpredictable few months, though. No real routine or pattern. Some days I am still reaching for my sweatshirt and closed-toed shoes. Some days it is hot and humid, and the skies open with rain falling violently on our skylights. It's good for the garden, I think. I can't wait to see what will bloom next.

I am at the pool, lounging on a chair and looking at the two enormous maple trees at the other side of the pool. They are so peaceful and full of life. Huge. Luscious leaves cover their trunks and extend down every branch, high and wide. The same trees I look at every summer, ever-present and stable, even during the most tumultuous period of my life in 2013. Look at the trees, I think. They were here before and they will be here after. Unless they rip them down when they renovate the club, I can't help but think.

Anything is possible.

"Come into the pool, Mommy," said then-four-year-old, cutting into my mental clutter.

"Try it," said my husband. I took off my pants, stepped in, and waded up to my waist. The water was heated, but I was freezing. Shivering.

My daughter jumped up on me and wrapped her legs around my waist and her hands around my neck. "Come on, Mommy."

I smiled as if everything were normal. Did she think I looked strange? I heard a familiar voice: a woman my age whom I had met at some point, socializing with another woman. Did they see me? They laughed and talked loudly, moved around freely, maybe donning hats and sunglasses, but their bikini-clad bodies were almost bare. Their kids splashed around us.

"You are so slippery, Mommy," she said. "I keep falling off you."

I was catapulted back to earth. Was I so thin that she couldn't grasp onto me? Or was it the slippery long sleeve of my suit? Did she have any idea how sick her mother was? What did her words mean?

I watch the maple trees and wonder what this summer will hold. I look down at myself. I have no idea what is going on inside my body. It is too complicated to understand, and I don't have the same instincts I used to.

My arms and legs are back, I notice, even a touch of cellulite on the thighs. My sun hat is smaller this year, and I go in and out of the pool, now with my four-year-old, not fearful of the sun, the cold water, or my energy levels.

Another summer and I am filled with gratitude. But my future is uncertain. I sit by myself and listen to the sounds of my family and friends surrounding me, like a blanket.

A woman I know recognizes me from across the pool, yells my name, and comes over to chat. "Want to grab a cocktail next week?" she says.

Why not, I think.

Sincerely,
Shanna

September 2015

Dear Professor,

When I walked into your class yesterday I felt the familiar first day of school jitters. Everyone turned to look at me, and I looked at everyone else. The class was on the 4th floor and brightly lit. I still can't get over how much more modern everything is than in my college days, with large tables, smart computer screens and ergonomic chairs.

This semester I am taking Introduction to Architecture and Interiors, which is one of the first classes out of the 15 necessary to complete the Residential Interior Design Certificate Program I enrolled in. I am a student again, at age 37.

When I started the program this past Spring, I looked at it as a new endeavor, something creative and exciting to do. I am already waist-deep in fabrics, measurements, floor plans, color schemes, furniture and dream houses. I know the lingo; I understand the field. I can see a world before me that I never imagined I would be part of. And that I am still not sure I want to dive into. Given my situation.

I sat down gingerly, quietly berating myself for being late, but then remembering that I would have been on time if it weren't for the traffic on I-95. Be nice to yourself, I reminded myself. I smiled at the familiar face next to me, a woman with impeccable clothing and short blond hair who was probably in her mid 60s and who had been in my class last semester. She always talked about design as her retirement interest, maybe a new career. I may be younger than she, but perhaps that is what this is for me, too.

Yesterday you lectured about furniture styles during the American colonial period. I have a minor obsession with colonialism and was immediately taken with the experience of the

Europeans in a new world building shelters and furniture for their most revered family members and eventually more ornate pieces to show off their wealth. How fascinating to look at objects that were once sat upon and slept in by people nearly 300 years ago. War heroes, homemakers, children, politicians. They have been dead for a long time, I thought. The craftsmen who constructed the pieces we looked at hand-made each one. All that skill and effort. They are dead, too. And life moved on.

The tombstone in the old colonial cemetery in my seaside neighborhood flashed in front of my eyes. Ann, wife and mother, aged 37. I think about her every time I walk by her grave. Where did she live exactly? What did her house look like? How did she die?

I have an internal dilemma about what I am doing and why am I doing it. After all, here I am – a 37-year-old woman, mom and former business executive with a Stage Four and potentially terminal diagnosis, getting a new degree and starting a new career. It doesn't make a whole lot of sense, yet I am continually drawn to it.

I walk around the streets in my historic neighborhood thinking about the families that once lived there, and conjure up ways that I would restore the homes back to their original style. I watch in awe as houses are knocked down, replaced by modern designs erected from scratch. When I visit friends, I think about how their houses can be expanded and renovated. Beautified. When we visit friends' waterfront homes, I long to have one of my own, to relax and dream in.

My husband and I search the real estate websites and have our pulse on the market as we agree that our house is getting too small for our family. Should we move, build, or expand? Should we buy a country house? So many questions, with no answers yet, but every year I wait for the universe to show me the way. Meanwhile, I spend countless hours taking care of our little colonial treasure.

It is my sacred place. Our first home. The place where I got sick and spent months recovering in bed and in the garden. The place where our kids grew up and became little people. The Rockport grey exterior paint with Blackberry shutters and door and White Dove trim. The large side garden with purple sage and yellow day lilies and tall black-eyed Susan's lining the path to the back. The L-shaped backyard with the play-set my in-laws gave us when we first moved in. The new adobe garden gate that I went to great pains to wind the old wisteria around.

I remember my younger daughter on the baby swing while my older daughter learned to pump her little legs on the big-girl swing. The photo shoot we did there when I was 20 pounds too skinny and bald. I remember the backyard crowded with the entire neighborhood a year later, when we hosted the block party. And the front yard filled with my daughters' friends for their birthday parties, as an ice cream truck pulled up to surprise them.

How could we leave this place? I want more space for my husband to work comfortably, for guests to stay, for the girls to grow into teenagers, for me to do my artwork and relax in my own big bathtub. More closets and storage for everyone. Are these good enough reasons to move and leave it all behind? Take on the stress? Given my situation.

I guess the point is, dear professor, that here I am in my child-rearing years, with a serious illness and an existential crisis, and insistently drawn to all things home. On a practical level. On an aspirational level. And on a spiritual level.

Truth be told, I know I would never have come this far without such a solid feeling of home and the comforts that have supported me in times of pain, joy and all the transitions between. And I wonder how to further this passion in my daily and future lives.

It's not as straightforward as when I graduated from college with a degree in Communications and Marketing. I got a job at a large corporate brand. I worked my way up the ranks. I launched new programs. Made more money. Navigated and achieved. Grew up.

Now life is more about being than doing. I am worthy. I am alive. No need to be efficient. No need for busy work. No need to do anything I don't want to do to achieve the next level. And the level after that. This is my story. It doesn't make much sense to me as I am going through it, but interior design keeps beckoning me in multiple ways.

Maybe what I am trying to do is my own interior design. I am cleaning my house, donating old stuff, throwing out waste. Designing new space in which I can thrive individually and with my family. I am aware of my every move and am truly living in my body for the first time. There is an intruder in my house, named Cancer, but we seem to be co-existing, although she constantly causes me pain and discomfort. When she comes too close, she scares the hell out of me. I need to figure out where in my house to put her.

So, I keep going to class, sitting quietly in my chair among my classmates, listening intently to your lectures, as the story unfolds.

Sincerely,
Shanna

December 2017

Dear Therapist,

You have been my therapist for five years now. You have seen me at my highest highs and my lowest lows. You understand what living is like with such a devastating diagnosis, and the uncertainty that comes with it. I can't believe that you have done what you are doing for me for hundreds of other patients. You are a rock – a gift from the heavens. You have been and continue to be my companion through the hardest years of my life.

My mom found you because she didn't know what to do with me. It was shortly after my first diagnosis, with Stage Two breast cancer. I couldn't stop crying. I would wake up late and cry in my bed, shaking with uncontrollable sobs. Then I would shower, get into clean clothes, and transfer to the couch downstairs. Before long I would have another episode. There was no limit to my tears.

My parents had moved in by that point, recognizing that I was unable to function. "Why did this happen to me?" I would wail. Over and over. My dad would sit with me for hours and try to talk sense into me. My mom went online and called all the cancer support networks. That is how she found you.

In hindsight, I realize that I was having a true nervous breakdown. I thought my cancer was my fault. I was sure I was going to die. As you put it, I was brought to my knees.

I liked you right away. You were wise and smart. You were experienced. You asked all the right questions. You listened patiently to my story. You nodded and showed sympathy, but encouraged me to think about things differently. You gave tons of examples of women who had beaten this, who had moved on, and I started to feel better. We planned to see each other regularly.

You would come over every week as I battled the Stage Two portion of my disease. We would sit at the kitchen table – me in my pajamas and you in your stylish outfits. I admired your beautiful shoes and scarves. Never a hair out of place. We would talk about the week's events: how I was feeling, what were my side effects. But almost always we got to the bigger questions. Of family. Of disease. Of depression. Of life and death. I could talk openly with you. You understood what I was going through. You respected my accomplishments but knew who I was at the core and how this disease was going to change me. We discussed it all, and each time, I felt better when you left.

After I recovered from that horrible year, you coached me on how to return to work. I practiced what I would say to my boss and my colleagues. And I delivered on my plan. After I started working again, I saw you once a month, and then not at all. You told me that you represented the "land of the sick" and that I didn't need you anymore. I wanted to believe you. That you were like a fairy godmother, and now it was time for you to go. But somehow, I knew that it wasn't going to end that way.

A year later you called me to check in. I told you I was still trying to adjust to my new normal, and it was hard. You asked if you could see me, and of course I accepted. It was August, and I was already feeling the pain of the cancer that had metastasized to my bones. I was trying to convince myself that it was a tennis injury.

You showed up on a hot sunny day. We sat at the table on the back porch; I remember my little one was screaming as loud as she could inside. I told you about the pain in my hip, and that it had started on the tennis court. You agreed that it was probably nothing. You told me that I looked great and that you were pleased with my progress. Then we said goodbye, and I hoped I would never see you again.

A week later I called your cell phone and left a message on your voicemail. "It is cancer," I said. I was sobbing. "Please come."

When you showed up, I was alone in the house with the housekeeper. She let you in, and you walked back to the family room where I was standing. I didn't look up. I was crying. "I think we should talk," you said. "I don't want to," I said. "I can't." "Come and sit down," you said. I did, and the floodgates opened.

That was years ago. We met weekly at first. Now we meet monthly, sometimes bi-monthly. It took the first year for you to convince me that I wasn't dying. It took the second year for you to show me how to live with the ups and down of progression, switching meds, and getting through the difficult medical appointments and scans. It took the third year for me to gain the courage to discuss strategies for sharing the news with friends and family and to go back to enjoying activities and life in general. You have been with me through every single event and emotion. I would be terrified to make this journey without you. You have seen it all before. You have no idea how much that helps.

Now I wonder what the next year will bring. When I go to your office and update you, you have a smile on your face, and you seem delighted when I say things like, "I planned a trip to Australia with my family," or, "I am getting towards the end of my Interior Design program," or, more recently, "I raised $24,000 in sales of my watercolors for breast cancer research." You looked happily surprised when I said: "'I want to tell my daughters what is going on," or, "Do you think I should go back to work?"

But how quickly it can spiral. I know and you know that it takes less than a second. If the cancer spreads to an organ, then what? Will one of my treatments make me so sick that I land right back in that horrible state of self-pity and depression? How will my cancer affect my aging parents? How will it affect my growing girls?

You always remind me that, at the crux of my experience, I need to live in the moment. To live with the uncertainty. If I have 10, 20, or more healthy years, would I want to waste them away with worry? I am a type-A worrywart, so this does not come naturally to me. I am trying to change my ingrained responses, but change is hard.

I *have* changed though. Slowly I am realizing that. You are the one who helped me understand that there is no point in trying to predict the future. You are the one who encouraged me to go on with my life – with the painting, the design classes, the tennis, the family vacations. You are the one who taught me to see that I am a new person now, one who is living out her dreams, despite an unfortunate situation.

Sincerely,
Shanna

April 14, 2019

Dear Reiki Master,

You are part of my tribe. I met you almost seven years ago when this hell on earth started. You have helped me to relax and let go. To stop feeling like I had to control life, and to truly experience and enjoy it.

I am laughing to myself because I know you would say it differently. You would say that a divine power connected us and that my experience is not one of pain but of joy. That I have been sent a lesson from Spirit, and that I must learn it and spread the message far and wide. That you are my spiritual guide, and that you have opened the doors for my learning and development.

My mom found you. I still have no idea how. I think from talking to another breast cancer survivor who claimed that doing reiki with you was the most enormous source of support she had.

I will try it, I remember thinking at the time. I will try anything.

For seven years, I have driven to your cozy house, kicked off my shoes, and run up your stairs. We would chat about what was happening in my life, and in yours. Then I would lie on your table, and you would tuck me into your warm fleece blanket and rub essential oils on your hands. I could hear soft music playing in the background. The next thing I knew, more than an hour had passed.

You would change from a human into a channel for the spirits above you. I am sure of it.

Your voice would change, and your hands would shake as you told me about the visions you saw and the messages for me from up above.

"Don't worry about the medical jargon," you would say. "Healing comes from within."

"Stay neutral," you would say. "This disease is not good or bad, it just is."

Once you saw a young shepherd boy sitting in the dessert looking at the horizon. That boy was me.

Once you saw an angel from the Dark Ages spreading hope and spirituality in times of trouble. That angel was me.

Once you saw a beautiful butterfly opening her wings and flying in the warm crisp air. That butterfly was me.

During each session, you would place your hands tightly on my chakras – my head, my heart, my stomach, and my feet – until the energy in my body was rebalanced.

Most of the time you would tell me I had too much energy in my head. That I needed to be grounded. You would hold my feet down until you felt like that had been accomplished.

"Stop thinking," you would say.

There are so many messages that you have delivered to me that have resonated so strongly and brought me to the next level of processing my disease. I have felt so comfortable leaving your house and so confident that I could do this. That I could live with this beast. And live well.

A couple of times I tried to share our relationship with friends. They would look at me like I was crazy. "What does she do to you?" they would ask. "What does she tell you?" I would have had trouble explaining.

You told me to visit your spiritual guide, up in Connecticut, which I have done three times now. She gives me messages so powerful that I feel peaceful for weeks.

I really believe that you two are connected to some energy field that we can't see.

I really believe that you are healing me.

I am not sure how. But I will keep coming to see you because I know it is happening. Subtly. A little at a time.

You give me books to read, philosophers to follow, places to visit.

You understand more about the universe than I do.

You understand why we are here and what we are supposed to do while we are here.

You understand what to do during hardship and how to learn to live differently. How to change perspective.

You have followed my story for years now.

You are not going anywhere and neither am I.

But spiritually we are going everywhere.

Sincerely,
Shanna

Have Faith and Courage

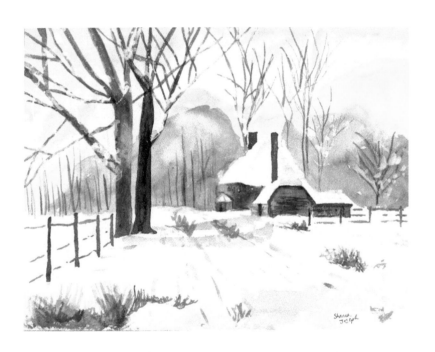

June 2016

Dear NY Doctor,

No one knows more than you do about how to manage this beast.

For years, I idolized you. I had heard so much about you — through the doctors, nurses, social workers, and receptionists at the cancer center. They talked about you like you were a demigod. I Googled your name and saw thousands of research articles, accolades, and interviews. The building that I visit every three months for my appointments is dedicated to you. I thank the universe every day that I am one of the lucky ones in your care.

You are a leader in the field. Until our first encounter, you weren't accepting new patients, so you were off limits for me. But I knew that you were somehow involved in everything that had happened to me since I was first diagnosed in 2012.

What serendipity that, in July 2014, I came in for my routine appointment and, instead of my oncologist, there you were. You probably don't remember the first day we met, but I will never forget it. I knew that my doctor was "on leave." My appointment had been moved around for six weeks before a receptionist called and told me that a doctor would meet with me until they figured out what to do with me. I was anxious, as I was having new symptoms.

I could hear your voice echoing in the hallway.

"Who is this?" Your voice boomed at the nurse.

She explained that I was a patient and that I was there for a checkup but also having new symptoms. "We weren't sure which doctor to send her to."

"What is it?" you asked, turning to me.

I told you I'd pulled something playing tennis, and that I'd had physical therapy for months, but it wasn't going away. "I think it's related to the cancer," I said.

"Point to it," you told me. I did. "No, you're fine," you said. "Go to a couple of physical therapy sessions here." And then you were gone.

Two weeks later I was back. The physical therapists at the hospital had done a series of MRIs and found cancerous lesions in the bones right where my injury was. "Well," you said, "it's probably a coincidence. If it weren't for the tennis injury, you would have been walking around like that for years, and I wouldn't have known or cared."

I rolled my eyes at my husband. Amazing that I didn't run for the hills. But there was something about your cavalier, know-it-all manner that I found appealing. It was a gut feeling. And when you checked my scar lines and listened to my heart and lungs, I saw in your eyes that you did care.

So, when you said, "You live in Westchester. How about I refer you to the best doctor up there?", I said, "Nope, I am staying with you."

"OK, now go live your life," you said. "You are a healthy young woman!"

That is precisely what I needed to hear. And that's why I think we are a match. I don't want to spend my time in your office going through test results, complaining about how I feel, and predicting my demise.

In March 2015, after my first progression, you said at my appointment in your office "'don't worry so much. I've got this. I have the perfect drug for this."

I know that you are ahead of the field, and I trust that you will prescribe the best medicine for me. "Ok," I said, scared out of my mind.

"And stop emailing me" you said. "I am too busy for that."

I emailed you the next week to ask you about my lab results. It didn't go unnoticed that within minutes you emailed me back telling me everything was under control.

One day I read an article about you. You were explaining your philosophy on how to treat patients with serious disease. "In my years of practice, I have found that those who look on the bright side live longer," you said. "I believe that attitude is everything." Mostly, I believe that, too. As do my most inspiring metastatic sisters.

Last month during my checkup, you tried to get rid of me again. "Why do you want to come to me?" you asked.

The way I see it, I had three options: I could go to a new oncologist up in Westchester. I could go back to my old doctor who disappeared for who knows what reason. Or I could stay with you.

For me, it was an easy choice. You are on the cutting edge of all new treatments, you understand the mind-body connection, and you care not only about me but about curing breast cancer for everyone. I will stay with you, please.

"I am not leaving," I told you firmly, and you nodded and changed the subject.

So here I am. You don't tell me much except "take this drug." You have tried to kick me out of your practice six times now. You probably spend more time talking to my husband about the stock market or basketball than to me.

But now, two years after our introduction, my gut is proving right. I am active, taking care of my children, and relatively symptom-free. The cancer is growing slowly, if at all. I feel healthy. Doctor, you are my lifeline. Hopefully I will be with you for a long time.

Sincerely,
Shanna

July 2016

Dear Nurse,

To you I was just another patient. I could tell by the way the questions rolled off your tongue, as if you had given them no thought. "Do you have any allergies? Is there a chance you may be pregnant? Did you fast for at least 6 hours? Did you hydrate? Where is the vein they typically go into? Did you use a hot pack on the spot?"

As you stuck the needle into that sensitive part of my hand, the only area still available for inserting an IV, I felt a warm shock, and the tears started pouring down my face.

"I am so sorry!" you exclaimed. "Did I hurt you?"

"Yes" I said, "but that is not why I am crying."

You nodded like you understood, but I wasn't sure you did.

You may have seen hundreds of patients like me, but I promise you, Nurse, you have no idea what it is like. The fear, the anxiety, the uncertainty, the raw emotions of wondering how much longer you will be on this earth. Because that stick, you see, is a symbol of what today is. Judgment day. Will I make it through this scan, stay on my treatment, and continue to live? Will I go on the vacations that we planned for this year? Will I get to take my daughters to their first day of 1st and 3rd grade?

On that hot, steamy weekend before the scan, I was like any other mother at the pool, slathering sunblock on the girls, begging them to finish their chicken nuggets, claiming the remaining umbrellas to put over my lounge chair. I was moving around the pool deck fulfilling my responsibilities as mom, wife, friend, neighbor.

But the dark sunglasses blocked the terror in my eyes. The white flowing pants covered my bloated belly. I was nauseous. My face was frozen in anger. My lips were pursed shut. And although it was subtle, I felt a thin foggy veil forming between me and the world. It was growing thicker by the minute.

As the day went on, I spoke less and less to people. I was more and more irritable with every request the girls made. I retreated to my spot on the lounge chair, where an invisible glue kept me in a still, fetal position. "Leave me alone," I huffed to my husband every time he spoke to me. Later, he fed me cereal in a bowl for dinner. The last supper, I thought to myself.

The morning after the scan, I woke up to the blaring alarm. Snoozed twice like always. Dressed and fed the kids, packed the swim bags, dropped them off at camp. Drove an hour to my interior design class, honking at the large trucks that cut me off and watching the cleanup of an accident on the other side of the lane. Always traffic on I-95, no matter what time I leave the house.

I was late to class again. Everybody looked up and acknowledged my entrance, as usual. The teacher asked how bad the traffic was. I settled in my chair, opened my notebook, and looked at the images of poorly matched design schemes on the screen being discussed until I was just as appalled as the rest of the students. I raised my hand and engaged in conversation like everyone else, went to the restroom, chugged my warm drink and ate some snacks, chatted with my desk-mates, and engaged with the teacher. No differences noted, I thought. This morning I am just like everyone else.

I jumped back into the car and realized I had some time before I went to my results appointment. I stopped at a local deli and ordered turkey and Swiss on rye. Extra pickles. Then went to pick up some samples at a couple of showrooms for my final project. I observed myself. Still part of the world, I noted. Maybe moving a little fast.

By the time I left the showroom, I was speeding up. My heart was pounding, and my walk was turning into a run. I called my sister from the car. My speech was faster. She tried to distract me. Asked me what furniture I thought she should get for her foyer. I looked at the speedometer and saw I was going over 80. Slow down, I told myself, you aren't in a rush. I flew into the city and parked across from the breast center. Smiled at the parking attendant. "Good to see you," he said. He remembered me, but I didn't remember him. His face was blank like a ghost. No features, just a shape. I handed him my keys like I was walking in a dream.

Then I was slowing down. Practically pushing my feet one in front of the other. I got into the crowded elevator and leaned my head against the wall. The sound announcing the third floor pierced my ears. My breathing was getting shallower. Suddenly it felt like two large bricks were on each shoulder. I took deep hungry breaths and tried to get air into my lungs.

My husband was already sitting in the waiting room. Texting with someone at work, no doubt, his mind on the market. He looked at me when I approached him, stood up, and gave me a kiss. I sat far away from him and didn't say a word. He knew I wasn't angry at him. I always need my space at times like this.

Time inched forward. I took an Ativan with water. Watched all the people in the waiting room. I always check to see if I know anyone and if there are any new young, bald heads. Old friends who have grown thinner and weaker. I flipped through my Facebook feed. Looked at all the cancer advertisements and brochures on the table. The air was warm, and it felt like the oxygen content was low. The florescent lights glared.

And then, after what seemed like an hour, maybe two, an assistant emerged and called my name. Someone whose job it is to sift through the cancer patients. Get them settled and get them to the right places, you thought.

I am here, I thought. My body had risen before I told it to, and I was flying through the hallways. Looking for signs. Was the doctor in the meeting room? Could I hear his voice? Were they talking about me?

The office always looked the same. The rooms neat and tidy. All of you were in their places guarding the doctors who were hidden behind closed doors.

Now a different you entered, my dearest Nurse. I have known you since I was first diagnosed. You used to seem so clinical and so professional to me. You still do but now we are almost friends. We know a lot about each other. We are similar ages. Do you feel that huge wall between us, though, or is it just me? You are part of the team that is keeping me alive. I am a metastatic patient.

"So how are you feeling? Any new symptoms? Do you still have pain in your hands and feet?" Casual but targeted questioning.

'Scans look good,' she said casually looking at her computer. I perked up. And took a long deep breath that I had probably been holding for two days. My husband did too.

"How are the girls?"

You have done this a million times. As have I. But the rawness never goes away. The panic. The fear.

We are always in the same room, dear Nurse. But we still live in two different worlds.

Sincerely,
Shanna

February 2018

Dear Boston Doctor,

I hide my right hand behind my back and cross my fingers. But this time I feel different. Calm in a way I'm not used to in a doctor's office.

When your fellow comes into the room to introduce himself and interview me, I barely flinch as I recite my cancer history:

Diagnosed in 2012 out of the clear blue. Surgery, chemo, radiation, hormone therapy, metastasis to bone, more radiation, more hormone therapy, more progression, switch to chemo, blah, blah, blah.

"What other medications are you on?" he asks.

I am on anti-depressants, anxiety meds, zinc, vitamin D, nutritional supplements to enhance my iron, antacids and probiotics for my belly, blah, blah, blah.

"What kinds of activities are you doing?"

Tennis, yoga, weight training.

"And how are you feeling?"

Fatigue, rashes, allergies, stomach issues, occasional nausea, anxiety. Otherwise awesome!

He smiles and says, "You're in the right place."

When you walk in, I can see your compassion and intelligence all over your face. My husband and I stand up to shake your hand, and then we all sit down to look at one another.

"I went through your history, and it sounds like you are doing well," you say. "No need to make any changes."

"Yes, I know that," I tell him.

I have had two good scans in a row – this has never happened to me before. My tumor markers are dropping, and my side effects are manageable. "I am here to talk about my disease and what you think about it. Going forward. I have a great doctor in New York. But I want to connect with a doctor in Boston in case..." My voice drifts off.

You nod and look down. Turn a little red. We both know there is a shelf life to these treatments.

"The drug you are on can last a short time or a long time," you say. "Next we would need to figure out if you are responsive to the HER2 positive set of drugs. If you are, it will open a whole new class of treatments for you, many of them in trial, without a lot side effects. If you aren't, we will know to focus on the chemo."

"I am terrified of chemo."

"You are already on chemo."

"I don't want more toxic chemo."

"Don't worry, they won't be as bad as you think."

"Are my days on hormone therapy over?

"Well, you didn't benefit much from that," you say. "Everyone has a different biology. What works for one doesn't necessarily work for another. It is a better bet to focus on other drugs."

"Okay, makes sense."

I take a deep breath.

You spend nearly an hour with us, answering our questions frankly. There is an ease in the way you explain things. It makes sense academically, and it feels like there is a path. I drink up your optimism. I've already been researching HER2 drugs and chemo where you don't lose your hair and half your body weight. Hmmm... if the drug I am on works for a while, it could be years until I am in real trouble.

My shoulders started to relax.

I remember when I was diagnosed with metastatic disease and had my first appointment. I was freaked out. I thought I was dying. And soon.

"You will do well," the doctor had said. "Don't worry."

But I *was* worried. I knew I wasn't supposed to Google it, but I did, and I was terrified.

Now it is years later, and here I am, strong and healthy.

You don't look worried. You look hopeful. You are telling me that I have options. That I have hope.

I am finally not worried, too. Or at least not acutely worried.

I am calm. It's as if we are talking about the weather. Assessing the situation and considering what to do if a storm hits. Or if it gets a little cloudy. Or, best case, if it stays sunny.

Sincerely,
Shanna

April 4, 2019

Dear Other NY Doctor,

When I checked my phone, and saw a missed call from the cancer center, I figured it was a receptionist trying to reschedule one of my appointments. I didn't even check my voicemail.

After all, I was at a day spa, and I had just finished a massage.

But when I saw another missed call, I started to get nervous. I looked at the voicemail and saw that it was 58 seconds. This was not normal. I quickly ran through my last two weeks. Did I have blood results coming back? Was there something they needed to tell me immediately?

I checked the voicemail and heard your voice. First you introduced yourself, but the message kept going in and out of reception and it was hard to hear. Something about your being a "nuclear physicist" and a "trial" that I was eligible for.

My heart starting pounding. What was this about? I was still at the spa and sat down on a bench to press the callback number.

To my surprise, you answered immediately.

I introduced myself and told you that I kind of got your message and was calling you back. "Does my doctor know about this?" I wanted to know.

You then proceeded to go into a five-minute spiel, starting with how sorry you were that I was battling breast cancer and how you hoped that I felt that I was getting the best possible care. It sounded like you were reading from a script.

Then you told me that you were a radiologist who was leading a novel study to see if women with certain histories have a type of cancer that expresses the HER2 gene.

"I know about HER2," I said, slightly annoyed. "I tested positive for it in 2014 and was on Herceptin infusions for four years.

I then tested negative for it in 2018, and my doctor took me off the drug."

"Yes, exactly," you said, like it was the most interesting thing in the world. "I believe you are still positive. If you are, my scan should prove it."

'Well, okay," I said doubtfully. This was my second experience with the word "trial."

Sometimes they can be lifesaving, I know.

But sometimes, doctors are simply using patients to test their hypotheses that may or may not make sense, and patients are left to deal with the fallout.

Last June, when I got the bone biopsy of the growing tumor in my left hip, I was lying down in my gown looking up at the interventional radiologist in the OR when he said something like this to me: "We are going to take a little more tissue from your leg so that the doctors can study your mutations for your trial. Can you sign on the dotted line please?"

He shoved a pen and a paper in my face.

I sat up alarmed and started crying.

"What trial?" I screamed? "No one told me about a trial!"

The doctor was in shock.

"Oh, I thought you knew about this," he said. "Just trust the hospital. We have your best interests in mind."

I don't know why, but I signed it. I had no idea what it was. The nurse anesthesiologist put a mask over my face and told me to count backwards from 100. The next thing I knew, I woke up in the recovery room, foggy and confused.

Fast forward to when I spoke to you, doctor, that day on the phone. I tried to picture what you looked like, how old you were, what your motives were.

I told you the story.

You reacted quickly. "I would never do that. I am telling you upfront everything you need to know. This can help you. If you are HER2 positive, you need to know. There are many drugs out there for you. This is a non-invasive scan with no side effects. You will get an injection of the radioactive material and then five days later go through the machine. Then I will call you with the results."

It sounded reasonable. Was I missing something?

I emailed my doctor immediately. "Oh yeah," he responded. "I think you should do it. It's a no-brainer."

Okay.

You emailed me with another form to sign. I almost signed it blindly again, but this time I read it carefully. It said that if the scan was positive, I would need a biopsy. You never told me about that. It also said I needed to get a brain scan as part of the trial. You didn't tell me about that either.

I called you immediately. "You didn't tell me about the biopsy," I said. "Or the brain scan."

You were clearly sorry. "Oh, don't worry,'" you said. "The biopsy is not for you. But you do need to get a brain scan."

Okay.

When we met in person, I was still suspicious. Firstly, you were at least five years younger than I. You insisted that I get a pregnancy test when I told you there was no way I was pregnant.

You were adamant that I would have no side effects even when I told you that I always fall in the less than 1 percent.

But I saw a glimmer of genius in your eyes. Something told me you were going to find out something spectacular about my case.

You gave me the injection and sent me on my way.

I felt sick and itchy for days.

I came back for the one-hour full-body scan. It was the same week as a CT scan to evaluate the pain in my left hip, not to mention my routine quarterly PET scan to see if my chemo treatment was working. I was exhausted and mentally drained.

When you called with the results, I was shaking. I had invited my parents to come over because I couldn't be alone, and they huddled around me. My husband was in the office and I conferenced him in.

"No brain metastases," you said to start. I breathed a sigh of relief.

"Your bone lesions are very HER2 positive. I told your doctor, and he is very excited. There are a lot of options for you." I could feel you smiling on the other end of the phone.

Wow, I thought. Just in the nick of time. I may not add new drugs right away, but how amazing to know that there are targeted treatments for me.

I had just found out the day before that my latest PET scan was good. And I had just found out the day before that the pain in my left hip was likely inflammation and not a break from the tumor. Could this be three good news calls in a row? After a year of fear and uncertainty? What if this is the beginning of putting me on the right track? Or, a little voice whispered in my ear, what if this is a trial that fails? That I am not HER2 positive?

That night I Googled HER2 treatments and the list was huge – and thought to be very effective. Herceptin was only the first one. I am going to choose to believe that I am positive and can benefit.

Thank you for getting in touch with me. Thank you for finding me and including me in your trial. It feels like you opened an entire new world for me. And that there is hope! For that, I couldn't be more grateful.

This letter is really a letter to research and science. Cancer is complicated. Treatment is custom. Timing is everything. Developments like these are exactly what we need to move the needle. Whether this is the trial that gets me on the right path or not, I just feel so lucky that I am part of the movement.

Sincerely,
Shanna

February 2, 2019

Dear Medication,

Here we go again. Welcome to my life.

My mom had come to the appointment with me. "I want things to look better," the doctor told us. Let's switch drugs. To something stronger."

Hello again, new medication. Hello to you, new side effects.

Now I must buy a new pill box to remember it all. Already on Xeloda. Lexapro. Ativan. Prilosec. Ibrance. And now instead of Ibrance will be Vernezio. Can I keep this straight?

The next day I spent six hours on the phone with the doctor's office and the specialty pharmacy company trying to get my prescription filled.

"Yes, my doctor ordered the prescription," I screamed condescendingly at the agent. "Why else would I be calling?"

"Well, they didn't do it right," she countered, just as condescendingly. "And they will have to do it again."

When the prescription was finally straightened out and in queue to be shipped, a representative said, "The pharmacist would like to speak to you."

That's a new one, I thought.

A deep voice boomed on the phone. "I wanted to make sure that you know you are being prescribed a new drug called Vernezio and that you are familiar with all the side effects," it said.

I said breezily, "I know."

The voice informed me that nine out of 10 women who take this drug experience massive diarrhea. "As a result," it said, "we recommend taking Imodium with each dosage. In addition, there is a host of other issues you may experience, including low blood counts, blood clots, fatigue, infection, nausea, low appetite ..."

"Really," I said. I was zoning out.

When the medication arrived, along with a huge bottle of Imodium, I popped a pill – small, oval-shaped, innocent-looking – and put the Imodium in a back cabinet. Accessible, but out of view.

I was constipated for seven days.

I was also achy as hell.

Coincidentally, my friend in Boston was starting the same medication on the same day.

"How's it going up there?" I texted her.

"Awful," she replied. "I have had massive diarrhea and been vomiting with fever and chills from this drug. Had to stop it and will restart at a lower dosage."

Here I was, the one out 10 patients with a completely unpredictable side effect not even listed on the insert. There she was, the same woman who had no problems when she was on toxic chemo the last couple of years.

What the heck? How is it that these drugs can affect people so differently? But then again, why wouldn't they? How could a chemical, and a strong one at that, be received in similar ways in different biological settings? In women of different backgrounds, with different diets, different genetics, different medical histories, different tolerances? I can see how difficult it is for the researchers to assess medicines in trial.

So, I have a new approach. I don't read about you anymore, Ms. Medication. Because all you are is a list of 'possible' side effects that have been recorded in a large tested population. That is why there are so many of you. And I could, and very often do, get some of you that aren't even on the damn list.

So, I will get used to you, like I do with every drug. You and I will come to an agreement, and you will become part of my routine.

And when we part ways, I will make some sort of peace with the next drug and live with you again, in another form.

Unfortunately, I know that just because you are controlling my life right now, the results can be variable. So, do me one favor. Please attack the cancer. Kill those pesky little cells. Or at least get them to stop spreading.

Sincerely,
Shanna

TRAVEL AND EXPLORE

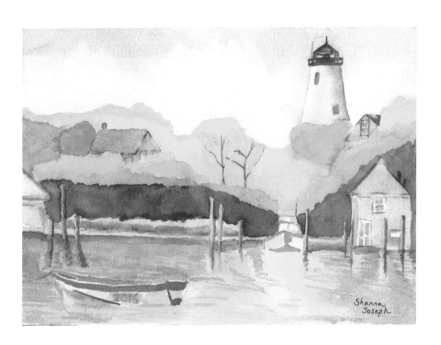

April 2017

Dear Wonder,

Since my diagnosis, there is something about being in nature that makes me stop in my tracks, take a deep sweet breath, and hold it for as long as I can. Then I open my eyes wide as if I can't believe what I am seeing. I blink a couple of times involuntarily. It is you.

I feel a longing to be close to you, and a deep appreciation of your powers. When I am with you, it is okay that I don't know the answers. You wrap your arms around me and reassure me that all is well. That my questions will be answered in due time if I trust the world around me. That not everything can be understood on a human level. That the world is as it should be, and it is beautiful.

We visited Alaska in August 2015, about a year after my metastatic diagnosis. The trip was originally planned as a thank you vacation for my parents, who had moved in and taken care of me during my Stage 2 treatment. But when the cancer metastasized in August 2014, and the following year turned into a rocky road of physical issues and emotional turmoil, the trip was postponed and we wondered if it would ever happen. It took months of adding to my suite of hormone suppressant medications and battling various side effects before I was stable and ready to get away. Our trip turned into a celebration of life.

My husband, the kids, my parents and I took a cruise up the inner coastal shoreline of Alaska, stopping at Juneau, Skagway, and Ketchikan. On my birthday, we went to the Mendenhall glacier. We had planned to get there by helicopter and walk on it with spiked boots, but because of the overcast weather, the flight was cancelled. So instead we stood in the national park across from the glacier and gazed at it. It was August, but I was wearing insulated pants, a windproof jacket, and my ski hat. The glacier sparkled. It looked like an enormous, bumpy ice skating rink that covered everything around it, vertically and horizontally. It didn't take much to imagine the entire planet blanketed by the same ice, devoid of any life. Endless cold ice, the sun shining on it from time to time between the clouds, shedding a blue cast of light.

A couple of days later, we cruised through Glacier National Park. The glaciers looked like waterfalls frozen in time, reaching as high as 100-story buildings. Blocks of blue ice layered one on top of the other, glistening in the sun, expanding for miles with trees poking through here and there. Every few minutes, a large chunk would break off and crash into the water, dissolving into thousands of shards – mini icebergs that were sharp like glass. The sound was so loud that I covered my ears to protect them.

This month, after a friend's wedding in Buenos Aires, my husband and I flew to Mendoza to see the Andes and explore the wine region. It was right after another turning point in my treatment: I had just been moved from hormone suppressants to chemotherapy pills. I was already experiencing the side effects, which included pain and redness in my hands and feet. I was thankful to have the chance to go deep into nature to heal my aching soul, which was terrified that the disease was progressing – again.

After we checked into our hotel, we took a walk around the property. The Andes loomed above us, majestic, but, to me, unreal. They looked painted into the background. There were layers of different colored trees, and then rocks so high that the clouds covered the top third. But you could still see the snow on the peaks.

How was this possible? I thought. These mountains had been towering here for thousands of years, and there we were, little specks of humanity vacationing below them.

These are the moments when I am sucked into nature, so much grander and more powerful than I am. These are the moments when I find you, Dear Wonder, hovering beside me, sucking me in.

Each time I leave an awe-inspiring landscape, I look in the distance and try to take a mental snapshot to remind me of a time when my life and my worries seemed insignificant. I am part of something so much bigger. For some reason that makes me feel better.

I add these snapshots to my collection of wonders. Skiing at Beaver Creek. The view of the Pacific in Cabo San Lucas. This summer it was Niagara Falls. Last month it was just the walking trail in my town. Last week it was the Long Island Sound during my neighborhood walk.

My husband and I have been traveling the world since we started dating. I have always felt your presence, Wonder, but I am so much more mindful and aware now of the effect that you have on me. I have learned to find you anywhere that is filled with nature and stillness.

Did I recognize you before my illness? Probably. But now I am paying more attention. You have taught me that nature will prevail. You know why I got sick and what will happen to me. I stand before you small and humble.

I wonder what secrets you hold about me and my future. For now, though, I will simply take note of your presence, wherever I discover it, and allow you to enrich my life and to comfort me.

Sincerely,
Shanna

August 2018

Dear King,

More than 2,000 years ago, you reigned. Your 30-room castle stood exactly where we stand now, overlooking the very valley we are looking at now. You lived in luxury and bathed like the Romans did. You were the ruler of the Jews.

Today I walk through the remnants of your castle. In and out of the stone-walled rooms. Past the old bathhouse. I gaze at the view, the rolling hills with palm trees and a fresh water source nearby. Then I follow your footsteps along the stones of the pilgrimage road up to the southwest wall of the ancient Holy Temple (the first one, and then the second one), where our ancestors came from far and wide to worship our one and only G-d.

Four years ago, when we visited Israel, none of this had been excavated. We saw the southwest wall and walked through some of the tunnels. But the castle was not yet exposed. At that time, it lay deep in the ground underneath a large parking lot and a bunch of houses. Unexcavated, like me.

This time, seeing the castle and its proximity to the temple finally let me grasp what the ancient city of Jerusalem looked like – and what it signified – all those years ago. It was the home of a community of sophisticated people – scholars and spiritual leaders, workers and businessmen – who were exiled from many lands, and who finally settled in their homeland, right on the mountain where Abraham and Isaac had started the Jewish religion thousands of years before that. Not so different from what happened during World War II and the subsequent creation of the state of Israel in 1948.

It feels powerful and personal to be standing in your castle. I can picture what you looked like: a gentle grandfather-like figure with fair skin, light blue eyes, long white garb and a cane. A clear and resonant voice. A sensitive soul. You were not tall, but you commanded respect and attention. You lived here with your family. And the entire kingdom of Jerusalem saluted you and followed your leadership.

I am your descendent. I do not know how we are related, but someone in your kingdom had a child, who had a child, who had a child, who had a child, and on and on until my parents had me. A trail of Jewish people. Over the generations, a diaspora of people. It is hard for my mind to comprehend the countless traditions that were upheld over all that time, as the world evolved – as cultures were formed, new languages were spoken, wars were fought, and babies born.

That holy chain of people somehow created the single solitary speck that is me. I have never met any of them, but I can learn about their histories and dream of what they might have been like. I am connected to every one of their lives.

Even as I stand where you, King David, once stood, I wonder whether my experiences here in Israel would be as poignant if I didn't have a terminal illness. Would I be as interested in a culture that was thousands of years old? Would I be as intrigued by the idea that I am connected to a chain of stories that goes back millennia? Would I be as aware that I am part of a long lineage, and that that lineage will continue to grow because of me?

Sincerely,
Shanna

December 2017

Dear Joy,

I have met you before. Many times.

We became friends when I was little. I remember seeing you at play dates, on family vacations and weekend outings, and during the summers at camp. Sometimes at school. Even when I evolved into a serious, studious type, I loved when you appeared – to remind me that I was a kid.

We stayed friends when I went to college and then became a young woman. Good friends. Those were my rebellious years, when exploring new territory, meeting interesting people, and partying like a rock star were the priorities. You were like a drug in those days. I would seek you out wherever I could find you and beg you to stay for the night. Then I would do anything it took to get you to come back.

As I grew into a responsible adult, you were harder to find. You were there full-force when I got married, and when I gave birth each time, but too often you were submerged under the demands of work, marriage, and child-rearing. You would still come around, though, if I made plans with you, to join us on a trip to the Caribbean, at a fancy restaurant to celebrate the week's end or my husband's bonus, or for a day at the park with the girls.

You were always a fling. You appeared like a fairy godmother for a drink, a meal, a walk, a night out with friends, a week's vacation, a summer of love. Always intermittent. Then back to the monotony of life. The hard work of life. The stress of life.

When I was first diagnosed with cancer in 2012, you vanished for two years. The skies were dark, and I was sure you had disappeared with the light. Even after the initial treatment, when I went back to work and my hair started growing back, I couldn't find you in the usual places.

Dinners with friends felt staged. We went on a couple of vacations and I felt like hell. My heart raced. I was weak for most of the day. I was self-conscious and scared. Although friends and family surrounded me, I was the loneliest I had ever been in my life.

After the cancer metastasized, the bottom fell out. I lost hope that I would ever see you again.

But about a year later, in 2015, you returned. I don't remember the exact moment, but it happened close to home. In my little town, of all places! Someone told me that I was smiling on the tennis court.

Then I went swimming with a friend in the Long Island Sound and felt this amazing rush of happiness.

Not long afterwards, I went to a concert with friends, and there you were again. Hidden amongst the crowd, dancing with me to the music.

Then, my sister and I went to see Taylor Swift along with 60,000 other fans. I am typically shy when it comes to moving my body in public. But this time, I didn't stop dancing for a second. I moved to every beat – every part of me – knees, hips, torso, arms.

That summer, I saw you at Rye Playland. On the Dragon Coaster, screaming my head off with my daughter. At the ice cream stand, scarfing down chocolate Carvel with my older daughter. Later, on a date with my husband in town.

I felt better physically. That probably had a lot to do with it. And I didn't have the stress of going to work every day. I got to see more of the kids and their amazing ways. Now that I was home, our lives were calmer than they had been with two working parents.

I remembered what it was like to see you, to feel you. With you, everything is brighter and more colorful. Louder and more melodic. I can smell the flowers and the scents of foods. I eat more. I breathe more deeply and slowly. I am present in my body instead of watching myself from the outside. I am not thinking about what happened five minutes ago or what will happen five minutes from now. I feel alive. I feel hope. I feel full, as if life couldn't get better. You are like riding a bike.

You began to come more often, unexpectedly knocking on my door and letting in the light and the fresh air. You have a way of making me forget my worries and the cancer.

Now I notice that you are living with me. In the room. Like a silent smiling companion.

At first I thought it was a joke. Why would a woman with metastatic breast cancer and a young family feel so light and happy? It didn't make sense.

But you kept following me. I keep finding you around every corner.

In the house listening to music, cooking dinner. Walking around the block. Laughing with the girls at book club, the moms at the kids' school, old friends, new friends.

Joy, we have become intertwined.

My kids ask me, "Mommy, why are you laughing all the time?" I reply, 'Would you rather that I cried?"

My husband mopes around after a hard day of work and says, "When do I get to have fun?" "Now," I tell him.

Today we went snorkeling in the Great Barrier Reef. It has been a lifelong dream to come here. To the other side of the world.

There we were in the sparking clear water. My younger daughter and I, side by side, snorkeling above the sea world below. Peeking into the cracks of the coral. Poking each other when we spotted the school of fat colorful fish pass below us and around us. Our fins and tubes bumping each other. Searching for a sea turtle. Swimming for so long that the lifeguard in the red shirt had to blow his horn and tell us we had gone too far.

My elder daughter and I, side by side, sitting on the soft sandy beach. Searching for small pieces of coral and seashells to bring home for ourselves and her classmates and teachers. The sweet breeze cooling us off in the hot sun. The crystal water lapping at our feet. Yelling to each other when we found a better one. A bigger one. A more perfect one. A pile of nature's creations on the shore.

My husband and I, side by side, looking at each other with love in our black Neoprene snorkeling suits. Laughing with pride that we made this trip happen. That we had crossed the globe with our kids to this little slice of heaven. Now we are literally soaking it in.

The four of us, hand in hand, swimming across the reef, pointing at the world below.

My mom and I laughing as she tried to breathe through her mouth because her snorkeling mask was on her nose. I couldn't believe she was going snorkeling. I couldn't believe she had flown so far to vacation with us. I don't think she could either. She was beaming with pride to be able to share in this experience with us, and so was I.

My dad and I gazing out the back of the boat on the way back from the reef, in awe of our surroundings. Both of us swam adventurously across the entire reef and compared notes later about the colors and creatures we saw. Both happy that we made this happen.

Next month I have my routine PET scan, to see if the chemo pills I take daily are still working. Every day here in Australia I rub my hands with three different creams to soothe the dry skin and cuts I have as a side effects of the chemo. I try to think about it as a chore. Like I am brushing my teeth.

I am not feeling confident about the scan. One of my tumor markers is starting to go up. This may mean something or it may mean nothing. I know all these drugs have a shelf life.

You will disappear for a little while as I get through the testing, doctor appointments, potential drug changes, and new side effects. Then, hopefully, you will return, and I will continue to see you as often as I have been seeing you. I really enjoy your company.

Sincerely,
Shanna

April 2018

Dear Garden,

This was one of the longest New York winters I can remember. Each day I would wake up with a chill in my bones and drink hot tea to try and soothe it. For months, there was a cold damp in the air that hung over us like a wet towel. The sky was grey and the ground was brown. The flu spread like wildfire.

I began to lose my way. I lost track of time. Of the days and the months. I felt sad and depressed.

We started to do less and watch more TV. Play on the iPad and iPhone more. We still cooked, but we ate less salad and fresh food. We went to bed earlier in the dark and then struggled to get out of bed in the still-dark morning.

Every day I would see the remains of you on the edge of my driveway. In the front of the house. On the side of the patio where my empty lounge chair lay covered with a wet tarp. Your evergreen shrubbery growing darker and wetter by the day. Your soil thinner and runnier. And lots of gaps where your perennials and annuals once thrived. The sprinkler knobs and irrigation hoses were more noticeable than ever. The garden gate to the backyard had barely been used in months.

In March, there were four nor'easters. Snow covered the ground and then washed away, covered the ground and then washed away.

At the end of March, we went to Montreal for Passover. I told myself that when we returned it would be spring. While we were in Canada it hailed. We bundled up and went tubing with the kids. Tried to make the best of it.

Then I traveled with my friend to Japan for 10 days. We explored city life in Tokyo before taking a bullet train to Kyoto.

The first morning there we took a cab to the Silver Temple. We were tired and looked for tea to wake us up. When we finished our matcha tea, we headed through the gates and followed the crowd into the temple.

I don't think I looked at the temple once. Because there you were. Finally.

A Zen garden. And suddenly that's what *I* was. Zen.

Lush green bushes planted meticulously next to one another up the hill and around the pond. Flowers peeking out where I least expected them. Enormous orchids and peonies in colors and varieties I have never seen before. Japanese maple trees and bonsai interspersed throughout.

The place was packed with tourists from all over the world, milling around with their cameras and backpacks. Usually this bothers me: I prefer to go to places that are local and less crowded. But today I was one of the tourists, and I didn't mind.

Because you were the most beautiful garden I had ever seen.

The path meandered and led us around the pond, over a small bridge, and up the hill on perfectly arranged stones. At the top, we looked out across the entire city of Kyoto. There were a few remaining cherry trees in bloom.

The air smelled sweet. It was calm, and my shoulders relaxed. My friend, who also loves flowers, was losing her mind with excitement. It felt so special to share this moment with her.

The transitions between the different parts of the garden were peaceful and natural, like they were leading me on with a whisper.

The path took us down more steps to a small forest of bamboo. Suddenly everything was shaded. The trees were like people huddled together.

Even though I was in a different country, I knew I had made it through the winter.

When we got back to our hotel, I checked the weather in New York online. It was in the 60s and sunny as far as the eye could see.

Sincerely,
Shanna

CREATE AND INSPIRE

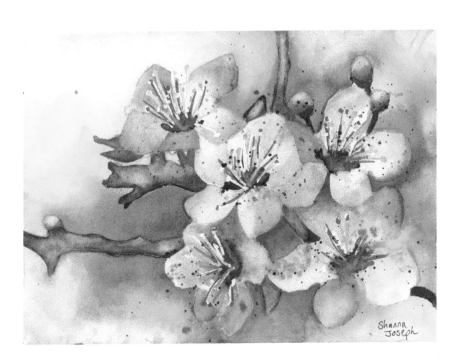

Shanna
Joseph

January 2018

Dear Watercolor,

I am not sure what drew me to you, but my gut told me that I must paint. Now. And with watercolors.

I loved making art when I was a child. I took almost every art elective in high school. Then I minored in Fine Arts in college. I had my own studio there, a small room that wasn't being used in the apartment I shared with my friends. I drew with pencils and pastels – portraits, figures, the occasional vase of flowers. Supplies were strewn around, and my works-in-progress hung on the walls.

On weekends, I would wander around Philadelphia visiting art galleries and museums. I spent a semester in Europe studying art history and exploring what felt like every art museum on the continent. I was obsessed; I couldn't get enough. I think art became a filter that made the world more beautiful and tolerable for me.

After I moved to Manhattan, I took up oil painting at a famous art school in New York. I met some interesting people and had some great teachers, but it was hard to get uptown after work, and the toxic fumes from the oils made me nauseous. So, it didn't last long.

Then I stopped. For almost two decades, I stopped creating art. I stopped going to museums.

I don't know why, but my passion for art vanished. The more time passed, the less I thought about it – making it or seeing it. I was working. I had a young family. I was busy with my new life. Art didn't fit in.

After I was diagnosed with Stage Two breast cancer, my mom convinced me to go to the art therapy drop-in sessions while I waited hours for my appointments at the cancer center. The first time I went, I looked around at all the paints, pastels, and pencils on the shelves. I had no idea what to do with them.

"I used to be an artist," I told the woman in charge.

She must have seen the lost look on my face. "Here, let me help," she said. "Why don't you start with this?" She handed me a box of crayons and a page that looked like it came from a coloring book. I sat there coloring inside the lines until my name was called and I left to receive my chemotherapy.

After I was diagnosed with Stage Four, I was flipping mindlessly through the local continuing education catalog when the watercolor class caught my eye. Something about "learn a new technique that is expressive and free." There were examples of landscapes and other natural scenes. The pictures looked so alive and the colors so beautiful. I signed up immediately.

When I walked in on the first day, I thought I had made a big mistake. The room was filled with older women – the average age was 60, maybe 70. They were chatting; they all knew one another. It was a generic and cold space, with long card tables and folding chairs. Some natural light, but not much.

The teacher was Hope. She was the same age as the others. After introducing the class and the day's project, she came over to me to check my art supplies. "Wrong, wrong, wrong," she said, her voice deep and slightly aggressive. "Go back to the store."

I tried to follow the instructions and paint anyway, but I didn't know what I was doing. I didn't know which of the ten brushes I had purchased to use for what; I didn't even know how to hold the brush. At the end of the class we hung up our paintings for a group critique. Some of the them looked like they belonged in the Met. Mine hung shyly to the side. "Good start," Hope said. "Nice color, but too much water and over-painted."

It has been almost three years since that day. Every Tuesday, I have trekked into that room, despite pouring rain, torrential snow, blazing heat, or frigid cold. I spread out my supplies, listen to the day's assignment, watch the demo, and then work with my head down for three hours straight.

I slowly learned how to mix colors and lay an underpainting onto cold press paper. How to manage the water. I re-learned how to draw perspective. How to make the light shine based on where it is coming from. Hope taught me how to paint clouds, still water, waves, waterfalls, snow, rocks, barns, birds, people, mountains, trees, bushes, and flowers. Soon I developed my own style.

After a while, I started chatting with some of the women, in the kitchen when we were rinsing our cups, sitting next to each other at the tables, or as we reviewed everyone's work at the end of each class. They talked about their grandkids; I talked about my kids. They talked about their ailments; I thought about mine.

I never mentioned my cancer.

Sometimes, when I had to miss a class for a PET scan or a doctor's appointment, I would pay Hope to come over and make it up with me privately. I never explained why I had to miss class.

One day, Hope looked at me from across the room and said, "Shanna, if I were your mother, I would be worried about you. Your skin is yellow."

I shrugged, figuring it must be one of my medications. But she scared the hell out of me.

I stayed focused on getting better at painting.

When I came home each week, I would dry my pieces by the window for a day and then put them in a clear loose-leaf sleeve in my portfolio. I now have two full books of you.

There were days, weeks, even months in a row that I produced horrible work. There were days, weeks, even months in a row that I produced masterpieces.

One day in 2016, I posted an image of one of my paintings on Facebook. I wasn't trying to share it; I simply wanted to make it my profile picture. I was shocked by the number of likes and the comments I got. "Create an online gallery." "You are a natural. Stunning! Can I commission a painting?"

That summer I shared two paintings that were inspired by photographs: the boats in Central Park and the Ferris wheel at Rye Playland. "Uncanny! Amazing!" people commented. Friends from around town. Friends from college, camp, high school, years ago, decades ago. I felt like I was capturing their hearts.

In January 2017, I announced that I was going to post a painting every month. Again, the response was enthusiastic and encouraging. I saw someone tag a friend of hers. "This is the artist I was talking about," she typed. I got so excited to share my work. My sister helped me name each one.

Then I had an idea. I could sell them! I didn't want to part with the actual paintings. Those belonged to me. But I could make prints. I announced it on Facebook.

A couple of people bought prints. Everyone in my family, of course. But as an interior designer, I know that artwork requires framing and an eye for décor, and choosing is personal, sometimes requiring input from others. It was a tough sell.

So, I switched to printing my pieces onto notecards. I boxed up twelve cards, with envelopes, and wrapped it with a pink ribbon. I printed "Sincerely, Shanna" on stickers and put one on the front of each box. The cards show winter landscapes, summer scenes, flowers, moments.

Then I had another idea. "All proceeds will go to breast cancer research," I posted.

When I came home that evening there were a dozen orders. The next day twenty. By the end of the year, I had sold almost 100 boxes and raised nearly $24,000 for research. I couldn't keep up with the boxes, the orders, the packing, so I closed it down.

I donated all the money to the breast cancer research fund at my cancer center. When I told my doctor about it one day at a routine appointment, he was aghast. I handed him a box; I gave another one to his nurse practitioner. They loved them. "My daughter is a painter," he said.

By then, I was already working on my memoir and the title of this book came to me. Letters from the heart. With words and with art. "Sincerely, Shanna."

Some letters are accompanied by a painting that I painted with Hope in my art classes, inspired by my experiences. I hope you enjoy them.

I have thought about you and why you are so gratifying for me. Here is what I came up with.

For the first time, I have learned a technique that uses the medium (the brush, the water, and the color) beyond the intrinsic skills of seeing and replicating on paper. As a result, I have pushed myself beyond "realism" and am expressing my own view of a subject. An interpretation. A mood. A slice of life. In the process, I am using repetitive brushstrokes, which I find soothing.

I also believe that, for a type A personality like me, it is gratifying – delightful – to start with a mess of color and water and turn it into its own world. Like magic.

And let's be honest. I prefer you over oil painting because you are more manageable, with fewer supplies, and because you are non-toxic (although my friend thinks you smell like a wet dog).

Sincerely,
Shanna

P.S. Prints and notecards of the paintings in this book are for sale to benefit the Breast Cancer Research Fund (BCRF). Send me an email if you are interested.

January 18, 2019

Dear Certificate,

You are just a piece of paper. But oh, how much you represent. Especially now when I am struggling with cancer growth and progression.

Four years ago, I researched you online. Interior Residential Certificate at a University. What the heck is that worth? It's not even a real degree. And I would have to take 15 courses to get you. Is it some money-making scheme at the school? To suck me in and get as much out of me as you can?

But when I looked at your requirements, all the courses excited me. An entire semester to learn about color? Textiles? Furniture? How fascinating!

My first semester of the program was challenging, to say the least. I was overwhelmed by being a student again, with my bag full of textbooks, notebooks, and pencils. The teacher talked so fast that I couldn't keep up. The syllabus referenced weekly assignments, midterms, readings, three hours of lectures every week. I was lost.

"Just do your reading, review your notes, keep up with your assignments, and show up to all the classes," the teacher said. "You will be fine."

Right. I could barely understand the material much less retain the information. I couldn't even read my own handwriting in my notebooks.

And oh, those lectures. I found myself captivated by the information. And then confused. Then inspired again. Then bewildered. I wrote as fast as I could, and my hand hurt. I hadn't used those muscles in years.

Some of the weekly assignments were highly technical. But what did I expect? This was art school, after all. I had my rulers, my pencil case full of 20 different varieties, four types of erasers, pads of various sizes and thicknesses of papers. With each course, I added to my collection. Before I knew it, I had a package of fancy markers in all shades, a set of black pens in all the point sizes, and six different kinds of straight edges.

The director of the program told me I needed an architectural board. He said that I could pick up a barely used one from the sister of a woman in the program who had died.

I drove over that day thinking how strange it was that I was getting a board from a dead person. I had so many questions that I knew would never be answered. Who was she? Did she complete any of the courses? How old was she when she died? Did she have kids? Did she have cancer?

I met her sister in the parking lot of the real estate firm where she worked. The woman was in her mid 50s – pretty and put together. I handed her a check for $200, half of what I would have paid if I'd purchased the board new. "Come to my car," she said.

I couldn't hide my surprise when she opened her trunk. The board was enormous and thick; it filled the entire space. It took the strength of both of us to lug it out. It seemed like it was made of bricks.

"Wow," I said. "I had no idea it was so large."

"Yes," she said. "I knew I couldn't throw it out. This is expensive equipment."

The board had a smooth white surface, with an attached ruler that moved up and down on a sort of pulley. We carried it together and laid it in the trunk of my SUV. I had to push down the third row to make room for it.

The woman eyed the second row of my car: my girls' car seats, all their toys and junk.

"How old are your kids?" she asked.

"Three and five," I said. "This is going to be interesting, going back to school and all."

Her eyes misted up. She didn't say anything about her sister. I acted like I didn't know why she had an extra board.

"Good luck," she said.

I drove away thinking about the dead woman's board in my trunk. It was like I was driving it into a new life. Yet I couldn't help but wonder if I, too, would die during the program. After all, it would probably take me three to five years to complete it. And the statistical chances of living with my diagnosis were only two to three years. Who was I to have the board if I might not be able to finish the program myself?

I was taking two classes that first semester and almost killed myself getting back into the world of academia. I was on a drug that made me fatigued, achy, and nauseous. The traffic to and from school was a nightmare. The teachers were strict and unrelenting. My car became a pile of junk as I started amassing samples of carpeting, tiles, paint samples, and piles of design magazines for my weekly assignments. I kept the board in my trunk because it was too heavy to lug back and forth into the house. But my textbooks made their way to our bedroom. And when I had large projects, I took over the kitchen table with my stuff. This program was going to consume my life.

I got an A in both classes. But I decided that taking two courses a semester would be too much. One class a semester would leave me some time to focus on the kids and my disease. Maybe I wouldn't get so stressed out about the program.

So, I did just that – one class every fall, spring, and then summer. I plugged along. Slowly and surely.

I started meeting people in the program.

Anna was a 65-year-old woman who had worked for her husband's company for years and finally wanted to pursue her own dreams. Cara was also around 60 and, recognizing that it was time to do something with her passions, had just designed her new beach house on Cape Cod. Camilla was straight out of college, with her straight blond hair, sports sweatshirts, and loud, perky laugh. Jamie was a young mom with a two-year-old, pregnant with her second child; she hadn't worked in years.

The woman I related to most was Claire. She had three young children and a dog and lived in a new house in Connecticut. She worked in marketing and had recently decided it was time for a career change. But she couldn't leave her job until she had her certificate and a foot in the design world.

I saw her running into class each week, her face drained. She always brought food with her, and we laughed that she had to eat on the go – there was no other time. She would work all day, then drive to class, then do the weekly assignments late into the night. She took two or three classes per semester. She said she was beyond exhausted.

She reminded me of me. Of me in an alternate universe. Of me if I didn't have cancer. If that me had decided to switch career paths, I would have killed myself to make the change in a way that was financially responsible. I would have been just as intense. I would have done it all.

But it wasn't me. I had quit my job and was on disability. I had all day long to do my assignments. Would I ever use my design certificate for something professional, I wondered? Or was this just a new hobby, another way to distract myself?

Sometimes before class, I would park my car near the main part of the campus and go into the cafeteria. I would pay $10 for my student lunch and wander around with a tray, surveying the choices. It was so loud in there. The students were mostly undergraduates, 18 to 22 years old. They would sit in large groups, girls on one side, boys on the other. I heard them making plans for the weekend, talking about their sports games, comparing study notes, complaining about upcoming exams. They would laugh boisterously and call to one another across the room. Their cell phones were multi-colored with different gadgets attached and always on the table right next to their food trays.

I was so intrigued by these students. I would sit by myself in a little booth and watch them. I would think back to my days in college and wonder if I had as much spunk and energy as they did. They had structure and a degree to get, paid for by their parents. Their social life ruled. They were happy and carefree, strong and healthy. They didn't have a clue what lay ahead of them. And they didn't care.

This last semester has been the most challenging of all. I was determined to finish the program. I had two courses left – hard ones. Each was offered only in the Fall, and I made the decision to take both instead of spreading them out and waiting another year to graduate.

One of the classes was the history of interiors. It brought me straight back to my college days. The professor would put up slides of furniture and tell us the date, the style, the details, the maker. We would scribble as much as we could in our notebooks. She started with ancient Egypt and proceeded until modern times. Really, she was teaching us the history of the world. How else could we comprehend the context? How could we understand the gilded furniture of the French monarchy without knowing its lineage and what was going on in Europe in the 18th and 19th centuries?

We went on class trips together. To the Met, twice. To historical homes in the Hudson Valley.

I crammed all the information into my head. I made time-lines and drew pictures in my notebook. I read at home. I thought about what it must have been like to live in every one of those time periods. My brain swam with new knowledge.

The students grumbled about how hard it was. I was determined to get through. It was all I talked about at home. "Did you know that in ninth-century China everyone in a family slept together in one bed?' I asked my husband.

I had to write a paper and do a 15-minute presentation in front of the class. I had to take a midterm and a final. I got an A in the class.

The second course was my last design studio class. For my final project, I had to design a 5,000-square foot loft in Chelsea. We were given an actual space and had to put up all the walls and design the kitchen, bathrooms, bedrooms, all the living spaces for a family – complete with built-in construction dimensions, AutoCAD drawings, images of vertical elevations, boards of materials, and pictures of the furniture we selected.

Each week we learned about different techniques that would help us. Halfway through, we brought our boards to class for a working session. I had my vision for the style and furniture. I thought I was on the right path.

Then, a week before it was due, my teacher ripped my project apart. She was not nice about it. Apparently, everything had been done wrong. I had to fix about a million things. She said that if I turned the work in as it was, I wouldn't get a good grade. I was almost in tears.

I thought it was unfair that she had saved all this feedback until the last minute. I tried to confront her but she was a wall.

That week I worked around the clock. My presentation was on the very last day. My last time driving to campus. My last time standing in front of a class and discussing a design.

I saw the teacher in the back of the room. She was smiling. I got an A- in the class.

Two weeks later a letter arrived from the director of the program. It said: "Congratulations to you, Shanna, for a job well done. You have succeeded in completing your Residential Design Certificate and will be receiving it in the mail shortly…"

Attached was my transcript. A list of all the classes I had taken over three and a half years. All As, except for two A-minuses.

And so, certificate, you are proof of what I accomplished. I made a career change. I went to art school! I worked through a very difficult program. I learned a ton. I have new skills. New contacts. New tools!

I have no idea what I will do with you, but that is not the point. You will always hang on my wall. To remind me – and my family – that you can always make a change. No matter what. In any circumstance. That you can reach for your dreams even if they seem hard and ridiculous. And that if you focus and work hard enough, anything is possible.

Like serendipity, that night my neighbor from down the block called.

"Did you finish that design program yet?" she asked. "We are doing a major renovation and tearing out our entire second floor. Can you be my designer?"

I hesitated for about a half a second. "Sure!" I said.

Sincerely,
Shanna

April 16, 2019

Dear Client,

I always wondered what it would be like to have my own business. And you have made that happen for me. In my own little way.

We have been neighbors for years, but now we will be connected eternally. Because every time you wake up in the morning and get your boys ready, the décor – the entire feel – of your home will have been created by me, in partnership with you, for you and your family.

You "hired" me after I graduated from my program.

"But why can't I pay you?" you asked over and over.

"Well, I just graduated," I tried to explain. "I want to gain experience."

You pushed back. "But it's tons of work."

"I know," I said.

The vision started with a piece of artwork. I looked far and wide for something that would inspire you. We visited galleries, and I sent you choices.

Too modern. Too old-fashioned. Too plain. Too abstract.

I knew what you wanted.

The palette you had specified was grey, gold, aqua, and yellow. I had suggested adding purple, too. But how the heck was I going to find a piece that had these colors in one image?

And then one day I did.

It was a beautiful abstract piece by an artist I enjoy who lives in upstate New York. He paints with metallic colors and large brush strokes. There is strong composition and emotion in his work.

You loved it, too.

For the master bathroom, you wanted a modern but warm feeling. I picked a contemporary floor mosaic of Calacatta gold, which is a traditional marble stone with gold hues. Matching wall tiles and brass accents. A large white lacquer double vanity.

The boys' bathroom will have swirling art deco black-and-white floor tiles with a large cobalt blue vanity and black accents.

Next up: the boys' bedrooms…

I am having the time of my life.

Sincerely,
Shanna

GET LOST IN THE MOMENT

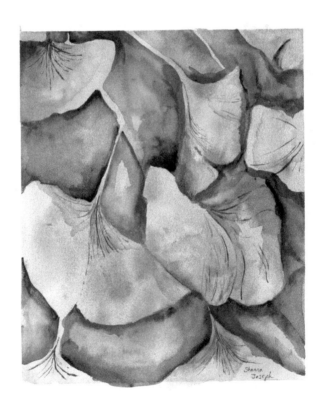

August 2018

Dear Favorite Singer,

It meant a lot to me to hear you sing at my 40th birthday celebration. Weeks later, I am beginning to work out the significance of the experience.

I first heard you when I was in college, in my friend's dorm room. Yours was a relaxing, indie sound. It was slow and moving. You were obviously talented at playing the guitar. And your voice was perfect.

But what moved me most were your lyrics. The actual words you were singing. They popped out of the melody loud and clear. You were telling stories that pierced me.

In college, I was conflicted about romance. I had had a series of love interests at sleep-away camp, as well as two serious boyfriends in my hometown, so I knew what it was like to be attracted to a boy. To get to know him. To get to know his friends, his interests, his hobbies, his moods. But college broadened the field; I met athletes and artists, city boys and country boys, men from different ethnic backgrounds. I wasn't sure what I was looking for in a man. I wasn't sure what I wanted my role in the relationship to be.

In college, I was also conflicted about friendships with women. I had had plenty of close girlfriends at school and camp, and I knew that unspoken awkwardness or tension was bound to arise. But now, on my own for the first time, I couldn't understand why a connection that felt so fun and fresh could sour, as friends interacted with other friends and jealously seeped in. My relationships were always filled with intense feelings, and college was no exception, as I connected with new groups of women, rushed and then pledged a sorority, studied abroad, and learned more about myself and my needs in friendship.

Favorite Singer, you were the beginning of vocalizing some of those complicated emotions. When I heard you, I felt like you were an old friend, there for me in times of change.

This song, one of your most famous, spoke strongly to me during my college years. I had never been to the Midwest, but there I was, still a teenager, away from home and immersed among new people. As I played your music and sang along with you, it made sense that I was singing about a faraway land.

To be honest, I pretty much forgot about you during my twenties. I was living in the city, so I wasn't driving around listening to music, and I was working hard, so I wasn't listening much to music at all. In fact, the only music I heard during that period was hip hop in late-night clubs and bars.

I also pretty much forgot about you during my early 30's. I was busy changing diapers, and my car CD changer was filled with the songs of Raffi and Barney.

It wasn't until I recovered from the initial breast cancer that I started to reminisce and rediscover music. I went back to the beginning, to the endless soundtracks of the '80s, from Billy Joel and Bon Jovi, to Madonna and Michael Jackson, to Wilson Philips and Debbie Gibson. These musicians were the backdrop of a carefree childhood, and their upbeat melodies warmed my heart.

Then I revisited the grungy soundtrack of my high school years – Pearl Jam, Nirvana, Smashing Pumpkins, Live, Matthew Sweet – when I rebelled against the fluorescent colors of my youth and changed my wardrobe to Doc Martens and flannel shirts. When my weekends included trips to the East Village and Roseland. When I started to have darker and deeper thoughts.

After a while, I decided I wanted to add more music to my repertoire. So, I signed up for Spotify and started to download songs. And more songs. I became obsessed with Pearl Jam, again. I listened to Coldplay, Jack Johnson, Adele, Taylor Swift, Maroon 5, Dave Matthews Band, Ed Sheeran, Phish, Pink. I memorized the soundtracks to Broadway shows like "The Book of Mormon," "Wicked," "Hamilton," "Beautiful," and "Dear Evan Hansen." The genre didn't matter. Pop, punk, rock, all of it. There was music in my life again, and it was growing. It was taking root inside me and making me feel alive.

And then I returned to you. With more focus. Your music reminded me of Indigo Girls and Joni Mitchell and the beautiful and intuitive female artists that my friend introduced me to at sleepaway camp. I loved your new songs just as much or more than the old ones I'd listened to with my freshman friends at college.

There were so many songs about the water, the beach, the beauty in the nature. You have put into words what I always feel when I am near nature: relaxed, carefree, and connected.

You sing about being with people and living in the suburbs and the strange interactions we have. You sing about going through hard times and then partying with friends to forget it all. About feeling hope and peace. Your words articulate what I am experiencing. They reaffirm what I believe. They reflect my life and make me feel better.

When I was going through the hardest parts of chemotherapy and radiation, and then recovering, I listened to you a lot. There was one song that I put on replay, and my eyes welled up every time. Were you singing it to me?

In the last four years, I have gone to more concerts than I can remember. Some of my favorite moments happen during live shows. There is nothing quite like rocking out and screaming the lyrics of the songs you know with the performer who wrote them. But whenever you were coming to town, I had some sort of scheduling conflict.

When my husband asked if there was an artist I would like to play at my 40th birthday celebration, I gave him a list: Pearl Jam, Sheryl Crow, Jack Johnson, Indigo Girls.

To his credit, he began writing letters, dutifully working his way through my list.

Then he asked me, "Who is your Favorite Singer?"

"Oh, she is the best!" I said.

We were in bed, and I Googled you to show him. I played him some of my favorites of your songs. There was a sparkle in his eye.

We quickly learned that you were born in Westchester and now lived in Long Island. The opposite of me! Within days, my husband had reached your agent and booked you for the event.

Then you were there, singing in the corner on that rainy night. Most of the room was mingling and drinking martinis, with a quick nod towards your beautiful voice, but I was mesmerized. Was that adorable, 50-something-year-old with a guitar really you? This time you *were* singing to me. No one else even knew who you were!

I see now that you – and music overall – have been the soundtrack to my evolving life. The messages I take from the songs I listen to and the feelings that music has stirred up in me have helped me know myself as I became an adult. Sometimes they've made me dance until I forgot my body; sometimes they've made me weep. They have propped me up in my battle with cancer. They have been a comfort, like a friend.

Sincerely,

Shanna

April 22, 2019

Dear Relief,

You arrived this week quite unexpectedly. Welcome!

I was sure this was it. The week I would be prescribed toxic chemo indefinitely. The gateway to feeling and looking like a cancer patient. The week I have been dreading.

This time I had come so close that I was okay with it. I decided it was going to be fine. I would wear the cold caps. I would get a port. I would get the treatment, and my cancer would go to sleep.

But there you were. First, with a text from the doctor late on Saturday telling my husband that the scans "were not bad at all" and that my husband should go forward with his business trip. We would not be making any major changes with my treatment regimen. My husband and I looked at each other in shock. You nudged us both.

Then you reappeared in the doctor's smile when he burst through the doors at the clinic and told us that the scans looked okay, that the bones were a little hotter but the lung spot is gone. Big news. So, we are back to bone only. "See?" he said. "The tumor markers aren't always reliable."

I realized that he was feeling you, too.

A few years ago, things would have been different. If I found out that my bones were hotter, I would have burst into tears. In fact, I would have been crying for days leading up to the scan and hours leading into the appointment. The anxiety has decreased. I feel you there.

Mostly I was relieved that there wasn't any major progression. I let out a long sigh, and I felt like I could fly. My heart rate slowed to almost-normal for the first time in a week. I could hear more clearly: the noises in the clinic, the nurses chatting outside.

I could breathe more easily. I felt young and fit; I wanted to run to the train station instead of taking a taxi. I think I was smiling.

By the time I got home, it was late and dark. Suddenly I felt physically exhausted from the full day in the city and emotionally exhausted as well. I could barely function. I moved slowly around the house, looking for food to eat, trying to get my pajamas on, talk to the kids, take a shower. It all felt like too much.

And then I remembered you, and I couldn't stop kissing my girls. Hugging them. Thinking about how grateful I was to have them in my life and to have more time with them.

After they went to bed, I became numb. I didn't know what to think, and I couldn't feel anything. I curled up in bed with a book and turned on some music.

Later, when I turned off the lights and snuggled into my pillow, sleep didn't come. I felt anxious again. Like I had that morning, before I got the results. My body tensed up. I tossed and turned.

You are good to me, sweet Relief, but because you visit me so rarely, the effect you have on me is strange.

There are the physical and emotional effects that I described, both positive and negative. Those I can handle.

What bothers me is how fleeting you are. In a few short hours, while I was trying to sleep, I felt you already leaving me.

Because let's be real. There is still disease in my body. Eventually I will probably go on stronger drugs, just not today. It still feels brutally unfair.

I spent an hour on Thursday discussing this with my therapist. "Why can't you find gratitude?" she asked. "You have so many treatment options available to you. You have a genius for a doctor. You have been going for years. Can you turn it around?"

I spent an hour on Monday discussing this with my reiki master. "The goal is to stay neutral," she said. "To stay out of your head. You feel good – let that dictate your emotions, not the tumor markers, PET scans, and doctor appointments. Keep living your life."

These are wise women. Their messages resonate.

So, is this what you are, my precious Relief? An ephemeral opportunity to look inward and think about what's going on more broadly?

I feel relieved that I have come to terms with accepting whatever treatment I will need to extend my life and be with my husband and my girls.

I feel relieved that I have gotten to a place where the scans don't feel as traumatic.

I feel relieved that my cancer is responding to treatment and is growing only slowly.

I feel relieved that I have such supportive family, doctors, friends, and professionals to help me digest all of this.

I feel relieved that I am still healthy and thriving, out and about every day, living a pretty normal life.

I feel you. Please stick with me.

Sincerely,
Shanna

May 2019

Dear Neighbor,

Did you know that I'm not supposed to be here right now? Don't get me wrong: I love seeing my daughter dancing gracefully around the studio. And what a great feeling to breathe in the fresh soccer-field air at 4pm on a Monday while hearing about what you're making for dinner. But this is a cosmic fluke. If I hadn't been metaphorically blasted out of my world in 2012, I would probably be sitting in my dark office this afternoon, analyzing how much people spent on their credit cards in October, while strategizing about how I could meet a deadline and make the 5:32pm train home.

"What a great backhand!" I encourage my little one from the side of the court, and she turns to look at me proudly. Where would my daughters be now? I think to myself. Probably camped in front of the TV, with a babysitter sitting next to them texting furiously with her boyfriend. I might have planned some activity or play date for them, but I'd never really know – or have the time to care – about the day's details. Were they tired? Were they whiny? Were they sunburnt? Did they have fun?

There are other moms like you whom I see on a daily or weekly basis, and I am starting to grasp what you do during your days. I can see how fresh ingredients are purchased, vegetable gardens grown, healthy meals prepared, new school clothes bought, houses cleaned, permission slips signed on time. I understand now how a child can be nurtured and shaped – into a social butterfly, an athlete, an academic, a kind person.

I am beginning to get the hang of it. I love having the house in order, doing things for my daughters and husband before they even think to ask, putting a structure into place around our lives that lets each of us move forward individually and together, and keeps everyone healthy, learning, growing, and, for the most part, happy.

I have a friend, another mom with whom I would have thought I had nothing in common a few years ago. Now she can practically read my thoughts, and I can read hers. We love to complain about how hard it is to squeeze in gym time while the kids are at school, even though we both work out at least three times a week. We like to wonder about what our kids are doing in class even though we are the only two mothers who sign up to chaperone on field trips. Wouldn't it be better, we laugh, if our husbands came home twenty minutes after our kids' bedtime than twenty minutes before? It would be so much easier!

Last week I bumped into a mom on the soccer field who I know envies me. How do I know? Because every time I see her, our conversation goes something like this:

"How are you?" she says with a guarded look, her two young children hanging off her. The bags under her eyes are heavy, her face pale and her hair out of place. I always think she looks put together, but up close I see that her makeup is melting and her shirt is wrinkled.

"Doing well," I say. "Heading to a tennis match." I am wearing my tennis whites. I look down and notice that my arms are fitter and tanner than they have been in years. My hair is freshly cut and dyed, eyebrows waxed yesterday. "How are the kids?" I ask. "How is work?"

"Can't complain," she says with what might be a cynical look. "I have been working all the time and the baby isn't sleeping. We should get that coffee. Wow, tennis – must be nice. Didn't you go to interior design school, too?"

"Must be nice," she says. "I saw your babysitter at pickup. You still have one?"

"Yes," I tell her. "You never know when you'll need the extra hands."

For a minute, I debate backing up and lying, dropping that I'd better go to back to work soon before the money runs out, or my husband kills me, or I get bored with being local all the time. To level the field.

Or I could tell her the truth. That I need my babysitter to pick up the slack on days when I feel like crap, and those can be any day. That I swallow a handful of pills with my lunch that cause GI and other issues. Or that I spend hours at my oncologist's office. I could show her the bruise on my left wrist where the nurses inserted an IV yesterday to draw blood and give me my treatment.

That it is my disability payments that keep me going so that I don't have to work and can take care of myself.

But I decide not to. I want to keep my distance and safeguard her opinion of me. I can see her self-doubt staring me in the eye: What was I thinking having the third kid? Will we ever pay off the house? Will I ever have time for myself? I want to make her feel better, but I let the discrepancy between our lives float between us un-rectified. "Let me know if you want to play tennis one day," I say as I smile and walk away.

The chronic reality of my illness is invisible, and I prefer it that way. Because I want to enjoy myself and my life. Not to have to explain details about my health that are nobody's business anyway. Not to be "that poor, sick girl."

I am not that poor, sick girl. I am the lucky girl. I am enjoying every morsel of my life. Because that's the way I want it.

Sincerely,

Shanna

Don't Wait for It to Happen to You

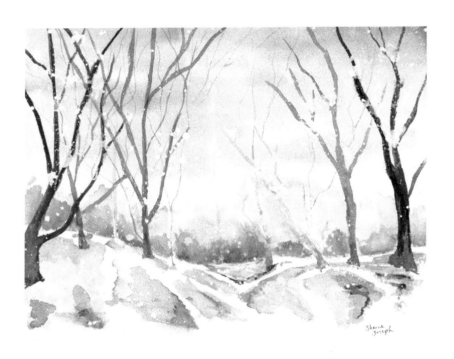

February 2019

Dear Mid-life Crisis,

You know what's funny? I have avoided you.

As I edged closer to turning 40, I think about what I would feel like at this point if my life had gone "as planned," a.k.a. no cancer. I get tastes of it by talking to my friends who are also turning 40. And it smells like a big mid-life crisis.

Some of their issues are physical. After all, four decades of living can catch up with the body.

Here's what I hear:

I am starting to get wrinkles.

I can't fit into my jeans.

My hair is limp, with more greys.

I have a new "condition" on my feet.

I need reading glasses.

I was hung over for three days.

I can't run anymore because of leg pain.

I also hear about stress and emotional issues:

I started Lexapro to help with depression.

I can't stop thinking and can't sleep.

I can't keep up with the pace of life.

My kids are driving me crazy.

Too much work and too many bills.

No time for myself.

Others are experiencing more existential questions:

My mom is dying.

My grandmother died.

Maybe I should have been a journalist.

Return to work or home with kids?

What am I going to do with my life?

Is this what it's all about?

I get to experience and think about all this, too, but for me, it is different. For example:

On the physical side:

I am starting to get wrinkles – YES!! I made it to old age!

I can't fit into my jeans – thank the lord; that weight loss was starting to worry me.

My hair is limp, with more greys – but I have hair on my head, and it is growing every day.

I have a new "condition" on my feet – well, I have toxins accumulating in my feet as a side effect that causes redness and swelling – a small price to pay for staying alive.

I need reading glasses – I have been blind as a bat since college. Welcome to the club.

I was hung over for three days – I have finally figured out how to have a drink without getting dizzy.

I can't run anymore because of leg pain – yay, more people who are limited like me. I can't pound my limbs because of risk of pathological fracture. Let's go out to lunch!

Now the emotional:

I started Lexapro to help with depression – Best drug ever, it works and good to know it's there if I need it …

I can't stop thinking and can't sleep – take an Ativan, for G-d's sake. I know that controlled substance sticker is scary looking, but trust me, you get used to it.

I can't keep up with the pace of life – the faster the pace of my life, the healthier I know I am. Finally, I can take on more.

My kids are driving me crazy – and I love every second of it!

Too much work and too many bills – oh well, what's important in life, anyway?

No time for myself – time is meant to be shared with family and friends. Don't you realize that?

And the existential:

My mom is dying – mine isn't but I am dying.

My grandmother died – and thank G-d she didn't have to witness me dealing with this monster of a disease.

Maybe I should have been a journalist – I want to be an interior designer, so back to school it is!

Return to work or home with kids? Both. It's all about balance.

What am I going to do with my life? Live each day to the fullest.

Is this what it's all about? Yup, and you have no control, so stop thinking about it, my friend.

Mid-life crisis, in some ways I wish I could experience what you should "really" feel like. But I also feel grateful that I already know the answers to the questions my peers are struggling with.

Like I said, I escaped your grasp.

I am an old lady in a body approaching middle age. I'm happy that I still look young. But mostly, I'm happy to be alive.

Sincerely,
Shanna

March 1, 2019

Dear Inadequacy,

I vaguely remember meeting you when I was in Stage Two treatment in 2013, and I was bald, skinny, and sick as a dog, at home with two babies. But that was a long time ago. If there are lingering memories of you, I have locked them away. Far away where they can never be accessed again.

With everything I have been through since being diagnosed with metastatic disease in 2014, for some reason I haven't felt your presence. I have been strong, independent, present. As my sister says, "if you didn't know, you would have no idea."

Yes, I have had side effects. Yes, I have had pain. Yes, I have been tired. Yes, I have had anxiety and depression.

But for all that time, I have managed to bar you. I have rarely slept through an alarm or asked for help from a friend for school drop-off. I have never missed a school event, even those annoying "come to school to do something ridiculous for 10 minutes with the kids" that the moms always miss by choice. I have never turned down a social invitation, cancelled date night with another couple, skipped an appointment with my personal trainer. I rarely missed a design homework assignment or a day of work last year with the designer. The refrigerator is mostly filled with food. The kids' schedules are always busy. The lunches are always made. The storage shelf is always filled with extra paper towels, garbage bags, and toilet paper. I have never flaked on anyone. In fact, I am the one who gets frustrated when someone flakes on me and we reschedule three times. You, Inadequacy, have not been there for any of it.

Don't get me wrong: I am so tired. I have taken many naps, snuggled on the couch under a pile of blankets for thousands of hours. I wear my pajamas during the day. Unless it is a workout day; then

I wear spandex. Or an errand day, when I wear sweatpants. Only if we're going out on a Saturday night do I wear jeans, a real shirt, makeup, and my contact lenses. My shoes are always comfortable and rubber-soled. I eat simple foods that don't take more than five minutes to prepare. I moisturize my face and apply eye cream every day. I am in bed by 10pm at the latest, and if I am not sleeping by 11pm, it is a rare event. I sleep late every weekend to catch up even more.

I noticed a shift with the start of this new year. It started with the rising tumor markers, continued growth on the PET scan, more meds and side effects, more Lexapro. Then the cold weather hit, and I lost control. In a way that felt different. More seismic.

It began with a chill in my bones in the beginning of January. I couldn't get warm. No matter what I did. No matter how many layers I wore, how many robes, warm fluffy socks, and slippers I tried. I bought a gravity blanket, and there was an ever-present pile of throws and a heating pad strewn on the couch. I closed all the blinds to keep the heat in the house and raised the heat to levels so high that our heating bills increased noticeably.

As the days progressed, so did my discomfort. I started asking my babysitter to get more and more of the groceries. I could usually be found on the couch in my pajamas and fluffy socks, under the pile of blankets, with a cup of hot tea in my hands. I didn't want to leave the house; I only did if I had something specific planned.

"Did you do anything today?" my daughters would ask when they got home from school.

"It's just the winter," I tried to reassure them – and myself.

Then it got ugly. We all got sick with various flus and viruses and stomach bugs that swept through the house in waves. The girls missed multiple days of school. My husband took Tylenol cold and flu meds so he could go to work. I couldn't move my body. My legs were achy. My nose was constantly stuffed or running, and my throat hurt for a month. Then it turned into a persistent cough. I was exhausted. My babysitter made daily trips to the pharmacy and kept our household afloat. Bless her.

I had too much time to think, and the thoughts I was thinking led me down a dark hole. Deeper and deeper.

Was I getting sicker? Do we need more help? Should I hire a live-in? Do we have to cancel our summer trips? Will the new house we purchased and the upcoming move in July be too much?

By the time winter break came in the middle of last month, we were all recovering, but it took longer for me. We went up to Vermont, and my husband took the kids skiing while I spent two full days on a lounge chair by the indoor swimming pool, reading and sleeping. I watched the snow pile up outside and listened to the wind blowing against the glass.

When we got home, I felt better. I wanted to go to the gym. I was ready to make plans.

But my most recent doctor's appointment was not so reassuring. My tumor markers continue to rise. There is still pain in my left leg. When they did an X-ray, they saw what may be a crack in the femur. They are investigating. If it is a crack, I may need surgery. Damn tumor eating away my bone.

I am scheduled for two PET scans at the end of the month. My doctor is talking more and more about IV chemo.

I am sicker. It is clear.

Inadequacy, you are like a dark black hole that I can easily slip into if I am not careful. You threaten me and my family with your width and depth, and your enormous potential.

I have memories of being sucked into you. I lie on the couch with my bald head covered in a red cotton cap; the TV is on in the background, but I am not sure what is on. I am thirsty, but I am too tired to get up to get water. My mom is at the edge of the couch rubbing my feet. I hear the kids laughing in the background, the babysitter shuffling through the pantry giving them their snacks. I hear my husband downstairs on a loud work call, laughing and being productive.

No one has said hello to me. No one has come over to give me a hug and a kiss. No one needs me for anything. No one even notices me. The days turn into weeks, the weeks turn into months, and the months into years.

I try to force myself to get out of my pajamas, into new clean pajamas at least. But what's the point? Depression sinks in. Sleep periods become longer. I escape from the tasks that define daily life. I am alone. You, inadequacy, are taking over.

Wait, I tell myself. That was 2013. I snap out of it. This is 2019. I type this paragraph fully dressed, sitting at Starbucks on a Friday morning across from my writing partner as we sit. I have made the kids lunches and snacks, packed them up, and driven them to school. My husband wanted to hang out since he is working from home today, but I am too busy. I need to finish this chapter and then go to town to get my hair done and pick up a tile delivery for a client.

Lately, the key has been living in the Present. Or the near Future. But no further than that. To focus on today and tomorrow. I am here, and functioning, even at a fraction of what I used to be. Even when I don't feel well. I am still making choices and enjoying life. I am alive and blessed.

I am back to that place of Adequacy. Adequacy defines me.

You are the opposite of that. You are scaring me. You are putting me on the biggest incline of the roller coaster life thus far. Toward what I fear will be the sharpest and largest drop.

Go away.

Sincerely,
Shanna

May 1, 2019

Dear Hope,

After seven years of living with my disease, seven progressions, countless days of being sick and sinking to the depths, of feeling joy and gratitude and the highs of life, I have found you. And as a result, I have learned how to truly live like ever before.

You were hiding deep in the trenches of my mind. I had to dust off the cobwebs and polish your surface until I was certain that you weren't an illusion. That you really were there.

Now I can see my reflection clearly in your mirror. My skin is smooth and radiant. My hair is long and healthy. My body is lean and fit. My mind is calm and alert. My feet are active and moving forward. I feel good physically and, more importantly, emotionally.

See you on the other side of this journey.

Sincerely,
Shanna

Now... Go!

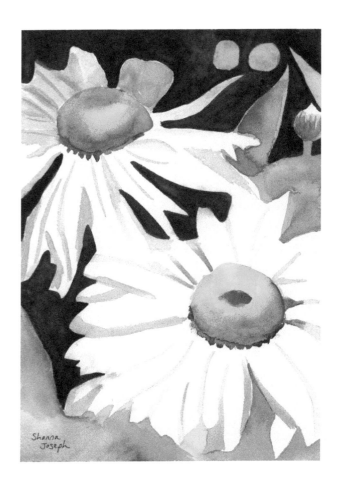

Dear New House,

I can't believe it is finally here. We are moving. Not far. Just a couple blocks away. But the significance of it is huge.

We love our old house. It was our first house: our venture into adulthood and the suburban jungle. It was where we raised our babies, made our first friends. Where I was sick and where I survived. It was where we built our garden.

It had been years of complaining about the little things. The original doorknob from 1938 that didn't close. The original toilet that always had issues. The handles on the French doors that were always loose. The crickets in the basement. The direct and awkward view into our neighbors' homes. The shoes and coats piled into the tiny front hallway because there was nowhere else to put them. My husband and I constantly battling for the single sink and vanity in the master bathroom. But we made do.

Then, over time, as the girls started growing, it seemed like we needed more space. Were we imagining it? After all, we only have two kids, and it was a decently-sized house. But the girls were always fighting in their small shared bathroom, and my husband had an uncomfortable work-from-home situation on Fridays, staring at the wall in his makeshift office in the basement. It was difficult to have guests stay with us since there was just one guest room and it was tiny and smack in the middle of the main hallway, with an adjoining equally tiny bathroom. Didn't do much for us since each side of our family is 20+ people. The dining room was also too small and only sat six.

I investigated adding an office onto the living room, pushing out the front of the house to create a two-level mudroom and master bath suite. But that didn't solve the guest room situation. Or my younger daughter's tiny-as-a-closet bedroom. The contractors told me it would take more than six months and cost more than $250K.

We could have stayed. But every year we found ourselves wandering into open houses and checking the listings online. None of them seemed right for our needs. Too expensive. Required too much work. Wrong location. And the years went on.

One day I had this idea that we could directly target just the houses in the neighborhood that look beautiful and see if the owners were ready to sell. Why wait for the brokers to get their hands on them? I wrote letters to the owners of two very cool and large homes nearby and dropped them in the mail. Both houses were at least 100 years old and had tons of charm and character on the outside. Hopefully they were renovated on the inside, but I wasn't sure.

Within a day, I received two phone calls. The first house was not renovated. Out.

The second one – you! – was perfect. In every way. And the owners were interested in selling.

You were built in 1894, one of the original structures on the peninsula. 10 years ago, you were gut renovated, stripped down completely, expanded, and rebuilt. The work is high quality. You are gorgeous.

The girls' bedrooms are large. There is a private guest suite. There is a big-enough office with shelves for my husband. There is a large dining room for family gatherings. There is a double vanity in the master bath. There is a bathtub for me!

You are next door and down the block from our good friends. You are across the street from the Long Island Sound, with waterfront access. It felt too good to be true.

The only thing that gave me pause was my illness. The last time we moved, I was diagnosed less than three months later. I worried that it was too risky to take on the stress. Was it even necessary?

The answer was yes. We are determined to reach for our dreams.

Within three months, my husband had negotiated a deal, including a close date at the end of the school year. I couldn't believe we had made this happen! We were doing it!

Three months after we made the deal, I had a chat with my sister about how great it would be to have her around. We could hang out, and the cousins would get closer. She and her husband were evaluating changes for their next stage of life, and the suburbs were appealing to them. The next thing I knew, they bought our house.

The whole thing was serendipity. I would tell the story to friends, and they would look at me like I was crazy. "What? You bought and sold a house without brokers?" "Your sister is buying your house?"

I am so excited. Now, just a week from our moving date, I am starting to envision our new life with you, in you.

I will plant baskets of colorful annuals leading up the walkway to the house, and maybe install gas lights along the way. The expansive lawn will be fluffy green, with the salty smell of the Long Island Sound lingering in the air. The front porch will be appointed with comfy wicker couches and lounges, and through the front door a new favorite light fixture will hang.

To the right, an airy living room adorned with artwork from all over the world and plants lining the wall of windows. A step up to the original dining room and butler's pantry, another era. The guest suite and sunroom waiting in the wings.

To the left, a beautifully designed brand new kitchen with every amenity imaginable. A cozy breakfast nook, homework room for the kids, office for me, large mudroom, powder room, and family room overlooking the Sound.

Up the stairs, a long hallway with all our bedrooms: larger than what we have now, but still close enough together.

On Friday nights, we will invite my sister's family over for Shabbat dinner. We will gather in the living room and dining area and eat yummy foods, and then after dinner the kids will go upstairs to play while the adults sit in the screened-in sunroom for after-dinner drinks and conversation.

My entire family will come for Thanksgiving and other events. We will light fires in all the fireplaces. Some family members will stay for the weekend in the guest suite. We will host huge barbeques for our friends. The kids will play soccer in the front yard and basketball in the street.

We will become closer with our existing friends who live in the neighborhood and make new friends with others who live there. We will say, "How did I get so lucky?"

You have been standing here since the turn of the last century. Did you have any idea of how much you would change the life of this little family? Of hope you could bring to an uncertain situation?

We can't wait to get to know you.

Sincerely,
Shanna

Dear Cancer,

You are not so scary anymore. You have been with me for almost a decade.

I have proven to myself that with the right attitude, medical care, and ongoing breakthroughs in science, I can persevere – and thrive – with you in the background. I have learned to live with you. And you have learned to live with me. I won't hurt you, and you won't hurt me.

Sometimes people die of you. But the population who is living with you is in the millions, and growing. Every month more medications are tested in trials and more are approved by the FDA. They are usually in pill form now; infusion centers have mostly closed. Rarely is someone bald anymore as a side effect of you.

With time, you will be a thing of the past. Like the Spanish flu. Like scarlet fever. Like polio.

Decades ago, I would have died from you, and quickly. But I was fortunate. My timing was good. I survived the uncertainty of you while you lost your grip on humankind. And started to fade into the distance.

Sincerely,
Shanna

Dear Family,

I will always be able to smell and feel what it was like to grow up with you in suburban Long Island, in that white split ranch, with the basketball hoop in the driveway and the play set in the backyard.

So much has changed since those early memories. Now we are all split up across the New York area. We have all moved multiple times and live with spouses, kids, dogs, and new belongings.

We have all grown up.

How scary it must be for you to know that your daughter, your sister, has Stage Four cancer.

I have tried to sugarcoat it. But sometimes it just comes out.

"I am dying."

"My hip kills."

"My skin is falling apart."

"I am depressed."

"I can't eat."

"I can't sleep."

The honesty of it all erupts in phone calls with you, in visits with you. You are among the only people I can be fully honest with.

But then just as quickly I change my tune.

"I am fine."

"We are going to Europe."

"I have four parties this weekend."

'I am taking the girls to five events this weekend."

"Want to come to Australia with us?"

"Want to come to the pool?"

It's the ups and downs of the disease. No one has seen it more than you. And my husband.

I don't want you to worry. But you are my support. So, it's hard to protect you from worrying.

I hope I have shown you that I am resilient and will keep fighting this beast for as long as I can. I am sorry to have put you through everything I've gone through, but I couldn't do any of it – I wouldn't be here – without you.

Sincerely,
Shanna

Dear Friends,

So now you know. I have cancer. I even published a book about it.

The secret that gnawed at me for so long is out. For so long I thought that if I kept the truth inside, I could go on as if it weren't there. But it is part of me. The same way my arms and legs are part of me. You can't separate them without changing the form of me.

I thought that if you knew the truth, you would feel bad for me. You would treat me differently.

I thought that if you knew the truth, you would be scared to death. About your own health.

I thought that if you knew the truth, you would talk about me behind my back. That I would be that girl.

All those things may be true. But I don't care anymore.

Looking in the future, I see many happy times together. Parties, travels, get-togethers with the families. Unfortunately, I see some terrible things, too. The death of parents, disease, loss of income and career digression. It is not going to be easy, friends, for any of us, and it is going to hit us all at different times and in different degrees.

We can't protect and control everything. Life is happening to all of us so quickly. Like on a roller coaster, just buckle your seatbelt, hold on tight, and go with it.

You can't predict. You can't hide. You can't make things happen, good or bad.

You can just observe. And stay aware of your surroundings.

Cry if you need to. Laugh if you want.

Hold onto one another. Ask one another for advice. Whine and complain. Compare notes.

And then wipe the dirt off your pants, get up, and start all over again.

This disease has made me different from you, I know. But we all have our challenges and our differences.

So, let's continue to respect one another and help one another. On this roller coaster called life.

Sincerely,
Shanna

Dear Husband,

Happy 15th Anniversary to us! In a couple weeks, we will be on a plane to Paris. To the French Open – bucket list! Then a couple of weeks later to Iceland to celebrate our anniversary once the kids go off to sleep-away camp. I heard it looks like the moon over there. There is nothing more fitting for us than to go somewhere exotic with a strange language and lots of beautiful scenery. Take me away.

It has been a long seven years. Since the moment the doctor announced, "You have cancer," until now, you have been by my side. The doctors poke fun at us because you accompany me to every single appointment. Every single one. Big or small. Even the ones I tell you it's not necessary. It is always you and me.

It has not been an easy road. The disease took away my health and a normal life for us at the prime of our lives. While the rest of our friends can focus on their kids and jobs, we need to focus first on keeping me alive. Not a small feat.

While the rest of our friends can focus on socializing and going to the movies and to dinners, we need to figure out first if my side effects are under control and if my immune system is healthy enough.

Somehow, we have made it work. In fact, we have done more than most people. We have put our minds to living out our dreams and not putting anything off until later. We have taken every trip that we have wanted to take. We have savored every moment with our family and friends.

And when the bad moments come, we share our tears, wipe them away, and turn on some good Netflix. Order in dinner and go to bed early.

You have let me sleep late, pile the sink high with dishes, skip my household duties, make a mess in the bathroom, steal the covers and take over the bed with my pillows. The house has been heated to my comfort level of 73 degrees despite your discomfort, and you have let my family and friends into our life whenever I desired.

You let me pick the order of our vacations, the house of our dreams, the flowers in the garden.

But we have designed our life together and will continue to do so. You have shown me that the end is nowhere in sight, if we have anything to do with it. To hold the faith, live in the moment, and be positive always.

We are doing it. I never thought we could. Seven years of living with cancer and we are happy and our kids are healthy. That is the miracle of our story.

Sincerely,
Shanna

Dear Girls,

To you, it probably feels normal to have a mom who has cancer. You never knew anything different. You were one and three when I was first diagnosed. You were three and five when I was diagnosed with Stage Four.

Although at times I shielded you from the details, with the help of my therapist, I have brought you along on this journey with me and with Daddy. And frankly, I couldn't have done it without your support.

You will always know what it is like to live with something frightening looming in the background. Even if you didn't quite understand what it was, the word "cancer" is scary and loaded. I am sure my fear and anxiety has filled the house with an energy that wasn't always pleasant. But you know what, girls? Although we would like it to be, life isn't always pleasant. You've had to learn that at a young age.

You will always know that Mommy had to take a lot of medications. My green pill box was constantly being filled and drained, filled and drained. I keep it on my desk in clear view and reach for it throughout the day. You know you are not allowed to touch it. You know those pills are keeping the bad cells away.

"Will I ever need to take those pills, Mommy?" you asked.

"No, not you," I say.

"Are these like the medicines I take when I am sick with a cold?"

"No, that is different."

When the cancer medicine commercials come on TV, I watch you focus on them intently. Looking at the woman who talks about the benefits. Listening to the list of side effects. Wondering if this is the same stuff Mommy deals with.

You will always know that Mommy lost her hair, wore a wig, and was very skinny and sickly looking when you were younger.

Maybe you were too young to remember, but you have pored through the photo books in the family room, and you know.

You ask me questions about it all the time. "Were you sad, Mommy?" "Did it hurt?" "What did it feel like when you shaved it off?" "What did the wigs look like?"

I answer each one honestly.

You will always know that I can lose my hair again, at any time. "That is why I grew my hair so long now," I tell you. "Just in case I need to chop it off again and build another wig."

We have talked about it so many times. "It's just a side of effect of the drugs, girls," I tell them.

"Well, we would rather you have no hair than be sick with cancer," they tell me.

You will always know that Mommy has a lot of side effects. Weird side effects. Raw and painful hands and feet. Bloody noses. Fatigue. Freckles and sun spots that appear at just the slightest bit or sunshine. Pain in my leg. Pain in my hip.

"How are your feet?" you ask me. "Are they getting better?"

I think you know if it's not one thing, it's another. That this will never go away. That this is my life.

You will always know that Mommy went to the doctor again today when I come home with bandaged up arms and wrists from the "shots." When I come home later than usual and the babysitter stays late again. When I come home with Daddy instead of by myself on a regular day.

You will always know that Mommy can't snuggle you on the nights of her PET scans because it is not safe for her or for you. And that she also can't snuggle you when you have a cold. Even though all you want to do is snuggle her when you have a cold. But you are okay with it. You are used to it.

You will always know that your mom tried her hardest for your lives to be like the others. With birthday parties, play dates, sports, school trips, and pool days at the country club. Weekdays jammed packed with activities. Weekends jammed packed with family and sports.

"What is my schedule tomorrow?" you would ask me every night before you went to sleep.

It makes me sad that you had to suffer all of this along with me. As much as I tried to diminish it, I know how worried you have been about me and how much you want it to go away.

"I will be okay," I always tell you.

The upside is that you know what it is like to see someone sad, hurt, and suffering. This, in turn, has made you compassionate, mature, articulate and independent in ways beyond your peers. Beyond your years.

Still, I wish I could take it all away. But something tells me that you will be resilient and happy in your lifetime, despite challenges that will come your way. That you will look back on your childhood with admiration and fondness. And you will know that I will always be proud of both of you.

Sincerely,

Shanna

Dear Future Self,

Do you ever look back and think that in your 30's you had a life-threatening disease? Unbelievable, right? Unfathomable, I know. Well, guess what? You made it. You experienced life's most difficult roller coaster. You built the strength you needed to live, and even thrive, with the Big C.

The truth is, it will never leave you.

You will always walk around wondering when the next bad news will hit. You will get tests for the rest of your life to monitor your disease, and occasional medication shifts to manage more progression. You will continue to battle annoying side effects, and schlep into the city frequently to alleviate them with more and more meds.

The truth is, there will be scary years and not so scary years. The cancer will go to your organs at some point. Because that is what happens.

You will think you are dying and lose 20 pounds. Then you will gain 30 pounds and wish you were skinnier. You will never know exactly where this is heading and when. What you do know is that it is never a straight line.

You will have months where you are so sick with side effects that you can barely leave the house.

You will have months where you almost forget that you have cancer again.

Your doctor will retire, and your nurses will get transferred to different departments. Your therapist and your reiki master will also retire. Your personal trainer will move to China. Your massage therapist will switch careers. You will acquire an entirely new team of support. You won't be as close with them or dependent on them as you were with the original team who saved your life, but you will learn to love and trust them, too.

You will travel with friends and family to every destination on your hit list. Some will be closer to home and more restorative like Maine, out West and down South. You will see the Taj Mahal at sunrise. You will ride a camel in Morocco. You will lie on the beach and soak up the culture of Bali. You will take a jeep through the camps of Africa and watch animals in their own habitats.

You will continue to exercise and play tennis and practice yoga. You will be forced to quit tennis and yoga because they are too taxing but you will take walks around the neighborhood with friends.

Your house will bustle with family, friends and neighbors. You and your husband will talk about buying a plot of land in the Berkshires and building that lake house you designed when you went to design school. You will also talk about designing a beach-front apartment in Miami, so you can have warmth and sunshine during the long, cold Northeast winters.

You will officially start your business and market it. You will have more clients than you know what to do with. Your designs will win awards in local and national competitions. You will be featured in magazines. You will train novice designers. If you want to. But you are not sure if you want to.

You may develop other interests and talents like cooking and playing the piano again. You may write another book. You will continue to read as a hobby.

Your parents will grow old. Your siblings will continue their life journeys.

Your husband will continue to work his butt off until he is happy with his career, and then start to back off.

Your kids will become taller and wiser than you. They will grow into more and more amazing beings and continue to surprise you with their resilience and compassion. Their talents will astound you. And you will be there to watch them grow up.

You will acquire more and more wrinkles. Your body will ache, not just from the lifelong medications, but from getting older. From being middle-aged.

And everyone will continue to rally around you for the rest of your life. With peace. With joy. With hope. And most of all, with sincerity.

Sincerely,
Shanna

Dear Reader,

I am not a public speaker, an actress, a comedian, or a cancer advocate. I am a reader, a writer, an artist, and a thinker.

This book is my forum and the way I choose to share my story. And it would not be complete without sharing the stories of the women who have guided me, and who continue to guide me today. They have touched my life in many ways, and I want them to touch yours, too.

When I was diagnosed with Stage Two breast cancer, I didn't understand the importance of support. I had my family and close friends and thought that was enough. I pushed all support groups away. I got through.

Then the cancer metastasized. Even though the same family and friends were there to help me once again, they could not understand my deepest feelings. I realized that now I needed more. I needed support from people who were going through exactly what I was going through.

Angela, born and raised in an Italian section of Boston, was the first woman to join my 'support.' She was introduced to me by a friend to be an inspiration, somebody who had been living with the disease for more than five years and was doing "well." Our first phone call lasted probably three hours. When she told me about learning that her breast cancer had metastasized to her bones, it sounded a lot like my story. She told me about the slew of medications she has been on and how with each drug, she would reach stability, and then the cancer would rear its ugly head, and she would have to start again. She told me that it was exhausting, but that if I had a doctor I trusted, a supportive family, and a positive attitude, I would live for many years with a good quality of life. Her kids were entering middle school; they had been in elementary school when her cancer first appeared. Since then she has quit her job, watched her kids grow, and gone to Italy three times. She told me that I would do the same. We promised to be in touch, and I hung up the phone feeling a little bit lighter. Now we talk pretty much every time one of us has a scan.

Kittie lives in North Carolina. She moderates a support group, which is a virtual monthly call that connects young metastatic breast cancer women from all over the country. It was about three years ago when my mom found the organization online and encouraged me to call. A single mom of two boys, she was diagnosed with Stage Four breast cancer from the start and has had no detectable disease for more than five years due to her ongoing treatments. Unbelievable! She told me this story on my first call, in her articulate Southern drawl, and I remember smiling ear to ear with the knowledge that this could happen for me, too. Every month she keeps track of our updates and checks in with us like a group mother. A community minded woman, she volunteers for many breast cancer organizations. She has inspired me to stay busy and healthy and have faith in the world and our path, which frankly is out of our control anyway.

I also met Tina through the calls. She lives in L.A. Like me, she was originally diagnosed with Stage Two breast cancer and went through the ringer of treatments. When the breast cancer metastasized to her brain, she was told that she could not have children of her own, so she and her husband hired an egg donor and surrogate to realize their dream of becoming parents. She told us this story on one of the group calls. Speaking in a soft, calm voice, she explained that with her background in film, she decided to shoot the entire journey. I think she is one of the most ambitious people I know. She made her dreams happen amidst the chaos of breast cancer and has inspired me to do the same. Although she has endured many procedures and the resulting ups and downs, her brain has been clear for years. We finally met in person when she came to New York for a breast cancer event. I remember being so nervous as we exchanged texts and described what we looked like and what we were wearing. When we spotted each other, we ran to each other and gave each other the biggest hug. It was like finding a long-lost sister.

Mara lives in Denver and is also one of the call participants. She was originally Stage Two breast cancer and has bumblebee tattoos for every year that she was in remission. In her strong, clear voice, she explained that she was working at her demanding sales job when she discovered the cancer had returned to her bones, liver, and lungs. She did a blast of chemo and was stable. But it keeps progressing, and she has switched drugs many times. She has a wonderful sense of humor. She believes that marijuana has helped her disease. All she does is open her mouth and I start laughing. She talks a lot about life *outside* of breast cancer, like spending time with her kids and potentially starting her own business. She has two young sons (one who's transgender). She has taught me that laughter is the best possible medicine, and that life's most valuable pleasures are found every day.

Kim, another call member, lives in NJ. She adopted her son after her original diagnosis of Stage Two breast cancer. But then, a couple of years later, she had a bad fall that broke her leg and revealed bone and liver metastasis. She has been stable on hormone treatments. She speaks with a feisty attitude and a Queens twang. Even before we met in person, she felt comfortable poking fun at people and making controversial comments. She is also not afraid to cry and show her emotions. And she can be hilarious. She is thoughtful and upfront about the issues she grapples with, like work, how to raise her kid while battling cancer, and how to balance her illness with her husband's gastrointestinal illness. She reminds me that we are dealing with complicated stuff, but that we are not alone. She also has taught me to be positive, always.

Anna is a quiet, beautiful girl who lives in Brooklyn. She was diagnosed around the same time as I was, but with Stage Four from the start. She has been on a stream of therapies. Kittie usually asks her a lot of questions and digs to find out what is going on with her, and she answers slowly and methodically. It has been hard to get to know her on the phone, and she hasn't shared much, but I have always been intrigued by her. My mom and I arranged to go to a metastatic conference in the city last year with her and her mom. We had a blast, bonding over dinner, sharing stories about our kids, and chatting until late into the night in her mom's hotel room. She has had some rough issues with anxiety and with her jaw, neck, and foot, but she gets through each of them like a champ. She has reminded me that, cancer aside, we are all individuals, and it takes time to get to know one another and form bonds, but once they are formed, they are there for life.

Jill is a sweet soft-spoken girl who lives in Washington, DC. She loves to shop and can often be seen in a bright Lily Pulitzer dress. She explained in barely a whisper on the phone what it was like for her to get diagnosed out of the clear blue sky with breast cancer as a young mother of two boys. And then to get re-diagnosed with metastatic disease just a year later. Just like me. Her cancer was relentless, and she went through lines of treatment quickly. From the outside, she seemed to handle it so well. She spent hours researching new developments and sought out opinions from all over the country. She tried supplements, exercised every day and spent countless hours with her sons. We were the only ones, besides Anna, of the group who kept our disease quiet from our communities at large. We bonded over that as we tried to protect our kids.

There are three other women who I have connected with outside of the calls.

Elle and I were introduced by a mutual contact at our old jobs who knew that we had the same diagnosis. We had worked at the company at the same time, never together, but we knew of each other. I can tell that we have similar personalities: we worked hard to achieve professionally, but we value family and balance. She was diagnosed with Stage Four breast cancer from the start; she did a trial in Texas to be "cured," which is not the typical standard of care. So far, her disease has disappeared, and she had gone back to working and running. She stays on top of her tests and all the latest research. She has taught me that there are many options out there – standard and experimental – and to network and keep an open mind.

Elle put me in touch with Diana, who also worked at my company when I did, though we didn't know each other. Now Diana and I speak weekly. She was almost dead when she was first diagnosed almost 10 years ago with more than 40 broken bones and a liver full of cancer. She had been misdiagnosed time and time again. She has had dozens of surgeries, radiation, and chemotherapies. She received an experimental breast cancer vaccine and has been NED (no evidence of disease) since. But she lives with chronic pain and discomfort. She is a talented jeweler and an articulate cancer advocate. I have helped decorate her house in New Jersey. We have gone to restaurants and museums in the city. We both love travel and art. We have cried tears of frustration to each other on the phone and given each other advice from deep in the soul. She probably understands me more than people who have known me for decades. When she first drove to my house and we met, she brought a bouquet of sunflowers. We hugged tightly. She defies all expectations and norms. We have discussed that her story could inspire an entire nation. I have never met anyone like her.

Elle, Diana, and I have applied for compensation from the World Trade Center Victim Compensation Fund. We are still waiting.

In August 2017, Diana joined a bunch of us from the calls on a weekend retreat for cancer patients at the New Jersey shore. I organized it. The accommodations, meals, and services were completely covered by the organization. It was the first time many of us were meeting in person.

On the first night, after we checked in and said hello, we decided to go out to dinner to unwind. It took us about an hour to get to the restaurant. It was raining, and some of us were in pain, some mentally out of it. Mara joked to a guy standing on the street that we were all Stage Four cancer patients and could he please put out his cigarette. At dinner, the bottle of wine went around and around; it didn't seem to matter that we were not supposed to drink. It felt like we could sit there for hours. The emotions of being together were overwhelming. We had only heard our voices on the support calls, and finally seeing one another's faces was powerful. We knew each other well. We all knew what it was really like to live with this disease. We laughed. We cried. We were sisters.

After dinner, we went back to the house, where we were greeted by a nun named Jo. She was employed by the organization; her job was to watch over us at the beach house. She guided us through an activity of painting inspirational quotes on sand dollars. Then we watched Tina's movie about bringing her son, Gray, into the world (which left us all in tears). We ate ice cream that Diana had made by hand. Then we all headed upstairs and passed out in our comfortable beds, with the ocean breeze moving gently outside the shutters. We were safe and at peace, even if for just a couple of nights.

I have one more friend, but she is no longer with us. Her name was Renee, and she lived in my town. The social worker at my cancer center introduced us because we lived in the same town and were being treated in the same hospital. Renee was doing well when I met her in 2014; she had been living with the disease for almost seven years. For years, we would go for a monthly lunch in town, and make fun of things we'd observed at the hospital, like the incompetence of the receptionists who planned our visits and the dramatic dynamics in waiting room. Then we'd get serious about what it is like to be sick with this illness while raising young kids. A former nurse, Renee was another mentor to me, ready with sage advice if I progressed or changed drugs. She was always optimistic. Even when she dropped 30 pounds after an experimental treatment. Even when she lost her hair again. She told me she was switching to another chemo like it was no big deal. Her eyes sparkled, and she squeezed my hand. "You will be okay, Shanna," she would say. "You will see." And I believed her.

One day, when I was walking into the doctor's office, I saw her. She was bald, with giant sunglasses, being pushed in a wheelchair out of the building. She was so thin and frail that I couldn't believe it was her. She had always worn a wig, but because we were at the cancer center, I decided it made sense that she wasn't wearing it. But still. Was she dying? I don't think she saw me. I sent her chocolates the next day. She texted me a thank you, wrote that she was on a new chemo and trying to get stronger. A month later I texted her and got no response. I Googled her name, and there it was: her obituary.

Renee was the first one of my friends who died. But it didn't feel like she was dying. Even when she was deteriorating right in front of my eyes, even then, Renee was living.

There are currently more than 150,000 of us living in the U.S. today. Living, not dying. Meeting each of the challenges that comes our way and forging ahead.

We are still here.

Sincerely,
Shanna

*Jill died in July 2018.

Acknowledgements

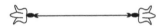

This book was the labor of love over many years. I would like to acknowledge the people who made it possible.

First and foremost is my husband, who insisted that I had a best seller on my hands. He was the first reader of the book and had amazing edits and ideas.

Next are my daughters who always knew that I was writing a book about our life in the background. Their constant questions like 'what are you writing about?' and 'did you get up to when I was born yet?' kept me going.

I met my editor, Susan Hodara, at the Hudson Valley writers' center when I dared to take a memoir course and start to process all that had happened to me. She was encouraging and sharp as a whip, and when I read my pieces out loud to the group I realized that I may be on the something here. My relationship with Susan has gone out of the room into a writer/editor relationship and she has read and edited every word of this book until I was comfortable with the flow, style and grammar throughout.

The meat of the book was written and rewritten over coffee every Friday in Starbucks in my hometown with my writing partner, Eloise Parker. We had quite a few laughs and pep talks as we surveyed the scene of fellow coffee goers which included two crazy men and the graduating class of the next door high school. Luckily, my car never got towed when I had nowhere to park but illegally but I was on high alert. Also, special thanks to the Friday morning barista who prepared my chai latte with almond milk and pumpkin loaf every week.

Special thanks to the beta readers/supporters who gave me final edits and the courage to cross the finish line: Sohita Torgalkar, Jennifer Furioli, Eloise Parker, Randi Spatz, Judy Delehanty and Linda Mitchell.

And finally to my loving family: my original six family members as well as the expanded clan with so many in laws and nephews and nieces that I have lost track. Thank you for being there for me always.

Sincerely,
Shanna

Biography

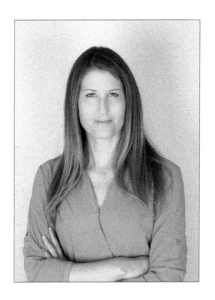

S hanna Joseph lives with her husband and 2 daughters in Westchester County, NY. This is her first book. The water-colors in this book are her own work and are for sale via email at shanna_joseph@hotmail.com. All proceeds will go to the Breast Cancer Research Fund (BCRF).